BEYOND WEIGHT CULINARY COMPANION

NUTRITION GUIDELINES, MEAL PLANNING & RECIPES

REZA YAVARI MD

INTRODUCTION

THIS IS a companion book for people who are on a mission to lose weight in a healthy and sustainable way for the long term.

The materials included in this book are available at our medical center Beyond Care and in our digital app BeyondWeight - available online. (beyondweight.com)

We decided it would be useful to make our guidelines and recipes also available to people at large who are interested in self-learning about culinary medicine.

These materials are generated and clinically tested over a period of 20 years. The average weight loss at our center is about 10% of initial body weight in 6 months and users of our app lose about 7% in 6 months. However, more importantly, our dietary guidelines result in long term and healthy weight loss.

We wish you great success in reaching your weight loss goal. Remember: reaching weight loss as a goal is different than other goals; *it matters how you get there.* Also, always keep in mind, *the number on the scale in not your goal; it is the consequence of your lifestyle change efforts.*

PLAN OF ACTION: FOOD SHOPPING

No matter what your goals are your refrigerator, your kitchen pantry, your car cooler, and your lunch box should be full of foods and beverages that are in line with your goals. Make a master list and go major food shopping once or twice a week.

- Buy fresh and seasonal foods; they are rich in anti-oxidants, vitamins and trace elements. The more colorful fruits and vegetables, the more they contain healthy flavonoids, lycopenes and other anti-oxidants.
- Buy fresh lean meats – preferably organic and free-range, as opposed to frozen or processed meat products.
- Buy cold water fish such as salmon, cod, haddock and tuna as opposed to fresh water or farm-raised fish; the former is much richer in good fats such as omega-3 fatty acids.
- When possible choose real cheese from a farm and not processed cheese made in a factory.
- Buy cage free and ideally local organic whole eggs and egg whites.

- Use herbs in your diet. They have no calories and contain minerals and other trace elements. They are good for you.
- Reduce the consumption of high-fat pre-mixed foods such as ground beef, pate and sausages.
- Try different spices, condiments, vegetarian spreads. They are usually low-calorie and add excitement to simple dishes such as baked fish.
- Do not buy junk food, soda; artificially flavored and colored products.
- Buy and eat seasonal and preferably local fruits, as opposed to off season fruits, canned fruit, fruit juice or fruit flavored products.

PLAN OF ACTION: COOKING

Cooking: Quick or Slow, cooking has to be methodical!

Learn how to cook and / or assemble quick meals. Also, learn how to do "batch cooking" so you always have leftovers for meals and side dishes.

- Plan and execute mindfully with a cool head and focused eyes; rushed cooking is often more oily or salty, has excessive energy-rich items like pasta, sausage, egg yolks, potatoes, etc., and does not necessarily taste good.
- Do not let yourself cook while you are starving; always eat a little something and de-stress before you start cooking.
- When cooking, play music or turn the TV to a calming channel, your food will taste better, and you are more likely to cook often if you enjoy it.
- Learn to cook simple; it is better to eat grilled meats, broiled fish and roasted chicken with a side dish of vegetables than say a pot roast or a complex saucy dish or a soufflé. The latter are often time consuming to prepare and could be very calorie-rich.

- Learn about the fat content of different cuts of beef, pork, chicken and fish.
- Choose grilling, roasting, and broiling over sautéing and deep-frying; the latter two methods retain most of fat in the meat and absorb the oils used for cooking.
- People who live alone often say "it is hard to cook for one person"; while that is true, do not cook for one person! Cook, pack and save the extra food (or give it to friends or family.)
- You may take an afternoon and relax while you bake a turkey, or roast two chickens or prepare a large stew or casserole. Divide them up into serving size portions; set aside enough for two or three meals in the refrigerator; freeze the rest. You could always microwave a frozen piece (at work for example) and add it to a salad or combine it with another dish. Be proactive and strategize.
- Use nonstick pans – for omelets for example, to cut the use of cooking oil or butter.
- Do not use recipes that require batter with breadcrumbs or flour. They soak up and retain oils - the combination of starch and fat becomes very energy-dense.
- Organize your cooking so you can save some for the next day; keep leftovers for future use (your freezer will soon have no room for ice cream!). Save the side dishes (streamed vegetables, sauces, etc.) to use in an omelet or a salad.
- Learn to use alternatives to starches like pasta or starchy vegetables such as potatoes. If you love pasta dishes, use them sparingly and as a side-dish not as the main plate. Obviously, rice, noodles and potatoes deliver less calories when steamed or boiled than when fried.
- Do not use too much vegetable oil such as safflower, sunflower or canola oil. These are rich in polyunsaturated fatty acids that may trigger inflammation and coagulation in the arteries. Olive oil is better because it has more monounsaturated fatty acids that are healthful.
- Buy and learn to incorporate into your meals low-calorie products that are healthy and add flavor, such as herbs,

shiitake mushrooms, garlic, soy beans, tofu, humus, ethnic vegetables, legumes and sprouts.
- Daily use of one glass of red wine for women, and two glasses for men, is shown to be cardio protective and prevent diabetes. If you do not drink alcohol, you can buy grape seed extract supplements.
- Use oil sparingly: Cook with olive oil or a natural cooking spray. Olive oil provides monounsaturated fats (the good fats) but be aware of serving sizes: one tablespoon contains as many as 120 calories! Use broth to sauté and moisten without extra oil.

PLAN OF ACTION: EAT

How to Eat!

Settle down and take your time. What you eat matters but how you eat matters even more: eat slow, chew well, protein first, protein second, everything else third serving!

- Again, be mindful of your eating: are you eating because you are hungry? Or are you eating because you are distracted and confuse hunger with stress or fatigue.
- Eat with peace of mind. Try not to eat on the run. Taste the food and decide how much of it you will eat. Be in touch with your senses. Use your recollections such as *"last time I ate this I got heart burn, this time I will not finish it"*. Be mindful.
- Avoid hunger; eat frequent, lean and small meals; always have a balanced approach. Do not eat fast absorbing carbs alone; mix them with other foods such as nuts, cheese, meats.
- If you have tendency to "inhale" too much of a calorie-dense food when you are rushed or hungry, be aware that regardless of the nature of the food you will over eat by the time you feel satisfied

- Do not eat the same foods over and over again; you will deplete your body of micronutrients, essential amino acids and fatty acids, which are present in other foods you are not getting. Variety is key!
- To lose weight you have to plan not to get surprise hunger pangs. If you get hungry always at a certain time like 3 PM, prepare a low-calorie healthy snack for that time or eat a bigger lunch, low in carbs but rich in protein and healthy fats.
- When you sit down to eat a meal, start with protein and fat then eat the carbs. The French eat crudités (like tomatoes, cucumber and lettuce in a vinaigrette dressing) before a meal to open up the appetite. If you do not want to stimulate your appetite go directly for the chicken or the beef; then try the side dishes – which typically have more carbs.
- Eat and talk about fun "stuff", engage in easy conversations that do not stress you. Socializing while eating slows you down. In Asian restaurants use chop sticks to slow you down. Learn to cut your meat as you go along eating as opposed to all at once (kids do that) and cut the slices in gracefully thin sizes you do not chow down. *You do not want to eat fast.*
- Learn to enjoy drinking water with lunch as opposed to sweetened drinks, soda or even coffee and tea (if you use cream and sugar). Some people believe that if you drink a lot of water before and during a meal, you will feel full and not eat as much; others argue that drinking fluids with meals accelerates gastric emptying and reduces the satiety effect; let your body be the judge.
- Use smaller plates so the portions look satisfying; huge plates and containers are shown to increase overall consumption of food and beverages.
- Always have low-calorie high-fiber vegetables such as bell peppers, and celery sticks in the refrigerator. A guacamole dip with celery sticks or bell pepper slices is a healthy, nourishing and filling snacks; you do not need chips for dips!
- Keep a food journal. If you are still losing weight or trying to address a specific problem like hunger and/or hypoglycemia,

you need to have a record of what you eat. If needed, you can consult a nutritionist to address your concerns.
- If you are a vegetarian, keep in mind that you may have to add extra protein to your meals; sometimes protein shakes or smoothies can be delicious additions to small meals.
- Stay hydrated: Water stimulates metabolism and helps detox the body; often times people mistake being hungry for being thirsty.
- Eat regularly: Eat every 3 hours to keep your energy levels high, the appetite hormone ghrelin in check and the satiety PYY signal high.
- Serving size: Calories per serving correspond to the calories in the serving size as defined on the label. These are often listed as a certain number of pieces, ounces, or cups. Look at the serving size and be aware that you may need to do some calculations. For example, if you usually eat 2 cups of chili and a serving is defined as 1 cup, you will need to double the numbers to get the actual number of calories you are taking in.

DON'T DEPRIVE YOURSELF: Follow the 90/10 rule. If you eat really well 90% of the time, you don't have to feel guilty about the occasional treat (call it a "dietary indiscretion" – nobody is perfect!)

POINTERS FOR BEGINNERS

Essential characteristics of all natural foods

- Constituents: Macro & Micronutrients

These are discussed in detail below

- Density: Generally denser foods contain more calories per serving; For example, hard cheeses have more calories per serving compared to soft cheeses

- Volume: Except for vegetables, bigger volumes usually indicate more calories; plant-based voluminous foods rich in fiber also provide bulk that helps bowel movements

- Water Content: Watery food items generally contain less calories per serving and are hydrating

- Color: Naturally colored foods such as fruits and vegetables are generally healthy; artificial colors are usually unhealthy

- Flavor: Naturally flavorful ingredients like herbs and spices have little or no calories and are usually rich in minerals and vitamins

- Cooking Method: Certain cooking styles are healthier than others; generally home-made foods are healthier, have less oil and salt than commercially cooked foods

- Measurements: It is important to have a good understanding of solid food and fluid measurements, portion sizes and serving sizes; many free mobile Apps are now available that convert various measurements

- "Free Foods": These are foods that have little or no calories and over-eating them is not harmful and at times satisfying

- "Functional Foods": These are foods – usually supplements – that are claimed to have health benefits or have medicinal uses

- Foods and Beverages with "Medical Warnings": People with certain medical conditions such as kidney, liver disease or diabetes are often given a list of foods and ingredients to avoid. Always ask your doctor if you have such dietary restrictions

- "Color Coded Foods": Green, yellow, red, and black colors are often used to simply classify foods for dietary plans. Green usually designates the best choices and red or black the worst

MACRONUTRIENTS & MICRONUTRIENTS

Macronutrients

Basic constituents of foods we eat:

- Carbohydrates: Starches and sugars in plant products such as grains, fruits or vegetables; all become glucose in the body; if not used for energy, glucose can be stored in liver, muscle and fat cells. 1 gram of carbohydrates is 4 calories.
- Proteins: All plant or animal proteins are made up of amino acids, which our bodies use for growth, repair but not so much for energy; if not needed, amino acids are eliminated in the form of urea. 1 gram of proteins is 4 calories.
- Fats: Include vegetable oils and animal fat; they are very efficient sources of energy and are readily stored in our body for future use; some are essential to our physiology. 1 gram of fat is 9 calories.
- Fiber: Usually refers to parts of plant foods that are not digestible; yet they are needed for general health including gut function and growth of good intestinal bacteria.
- Water: Essential for life, water also stimulates metabolism and helps eliminate by-products of foods and toxins in our body. Water intake is regulated by thirst, salt and fluid consumption.

Micronutrients

Essential foods we need in small amounts:

- Minerals: Refer to elements such as calcium, phosphate, potassium or magnesium – all major components of our physiology; trace minerals refer to those elements which are needed in minute amounts and yet they are very important for cellular function; these include zinc, selenium, copper among others and they are found in herbs and vegetables as well as animal meats.
- Vitamins: Refer to molecules that our body does not make and yet we need for healthy cellular function, growth and repair; they can be water soluble like vitamins B and C which are found in plants or fat soluble like vitamins A,D,E and K, which are found in oils and animal products.
- Anti-Oxidants: Refer to molecules including some vitamins that are needed in our physiology especially for damage repair, healthy aging and disease prevention
- Phytochemicals: Refer to natural colors in foods; these natural chemicals are involved in complex functions in health such as the immune response, disease prevention, recovery and slow aging.

FOOD CATEGORIES

Food categories:

Egg: A versatile, rich and common food; the protein in eggs is in the white and oils and therefore most of the calories are in the yolk; eggs are often used for breakfast but as omelets they make great, tasty and affordable meals; buy local farm eggs if you can!

Egg Products: Refer to food items that use processed, dried, powdered and frozen eggs. In general, these products are a common source of cholesterol in baked or processed foods; they should be avoided.

Meats: Refers to poultry or mammal animal parts rich in protein, fat, minerals and vitamins; they are usually consumed cooked or cured; animal meats vary a lot in amount of fat and thus the calories they contain. Portion and frequency of consumption are important if the choice meat is fatty; otherwise lean choices are considered good protein choices and may be consumed to satiety.

Meat Products: Refer to canned, cured or pre-made meats such as pates. In general, these products are high in fat and salt content and should not be used.

Fish: Sea or fresh water creatures include sea shell foods and crustaceans such as shrimp which overall represent a rich source of protein low in fats such as cholesterol; cold water fish have more omega-3 rich oils and are healthier than pond-raised or fresh water fish. Fish is a great low-fat source of protein.

Fish Products: These products – except for fish oil and some "imitation meats" – are not used in human diet (they are used in pet food and in fertilizers.)

Soups & Stews: Refer to mixtures of foods cooked gently in water or broth; they are common in most cuisines worldwide and can contain animal proteins and fats or made with just vegetables; they are easy to prepare and are affordable; crock pots and pressure cookers speed up the cooking times and make them more practical. These foods are usually low in protein content and calories in them come mostly from oil or fatty meats and starches used as thickeners.

Bread: This common staple in all cuisines includes breads, breakfast products such as bagels, or in sandwiches as rolls; or used in cooking such as in batter or "pockets" like dumplings or empanadas, etc.; these products are usually made from wheat flour and often require yeast to raise the dough; they are a major source of calories (carbohydrates which become sugar in our body) and are usually eliminated in most weight loss diets or restricted for people with diabetes; breads can be made from gluten free flours such as corn, coconut or cassava flour. See below for a comparison.

Baked Products: Cakes, donuts, muffins, cookies, snacks and desserts are not used in weight loss and diabetes diets.

Milk, Cheeses & Yogurt: Dairy products are versatile and common sources of protein and animal fat from cow, sheep or goat; they are now consumed more often as cheese or yogurt or as protein powder rather than milk (except when consumed by children.) Because most of the calories in whole milk come from fat, dietitians consider it as a "fat food" while skim milk is considered a "carb" because it is rich in lactose which becomes glucose in our body; overall dairy is a major source of cholesterol in Europe and North America; hard cheeses are very calorie dense and are often restricted in low calories diets or have to be portion controlled; Greek-style plain yogurt is now popular is a low-carb low-fat type source of protein and is often used in weight loss diets without restriction.

Nuts: Sometimes referred to as tree nuts, they include almonds, walnuts, pistachios and cashews and other less commonly consumed pecans, etc., are great sources of healthy oils, protein and minerals; because they are calorie dense their portions have to be controlled. Nuts are otherwise similar in their nutrition profile; walnuts and almonds are more studied and are clinically proven to have more health and disease prevention. See below for a comparison.

Seeds: Are similar to nuts in nutrition profiles; these include sunflower and pumpkin seeds and less commonly used chia, sesame, hemp and flax; they all have good oils and some protein as well as minerals etc.; overall, they have plenty of health benefits and should be in all diets.

Rice & Pasta: Cooked rice is a major food consumed by billions of people worldwide. All varieties of rice are rich in sugar and are therefore restricted in weight loss and diabetes diets. Some rice varieties such as sushi rice or Arborio used for risotto have more sugar and that makes them sticky. Brown rice has the same amount of sugar but because of its higher fiber content is considered healthier. Pasta is usually made from semolina – a coarse wheat flour. Noodles can be made from other ingredients such as buckwheat, quinoa, soy or cheek peas. Here too, all noodles are affordable sources of energy and have to be portioned or used occasionally.

Oils: They are divided into various categories: Saturated Fats raises cholesterol are generally not considered healthy; they are found in animal products, such as, meat, poultry, eggs, milk, butter, cream, and also in palm and coconut oils. Choosing low fat versions of these foods makes good sense. Trans Fats are found in hydrogenated or partially hydrogenated oils. These oils are created via a chemical process in which hydrogen is added to an oil in its liquid state, at high temperatures, to make the oil more solid. For instance, this is how a stick of margarine is made out of corn oil. These fats are commonly found in processed foods, such as, bread, crackers, cookies, pies, pastries, potato chips and are bad even in small amounts. Monounsaturated Fats lower "bad cholesterol" LDL levels and leave "good cholesterol" HDL levels intact. Olives, olive oil, and canola oil are good sources. For higher quality oil, buy "cold pressed" or "expeller pressed" and look for olive oil that is labeled "extra virgin" (first pressing) or "virgin" (second pressing). Other good sources of monounsaturated fats include avocados, nuts and seeds.

Omega-6 Fatty Acids are polyunsaturated fats that lower your total cholesterol; they are found in vegetable oils, such as, corn, safflower, sunflower, and most margarines. There is now evidence that consuming too much of these fats also increases inflammation in the body and may irritate the immune system. Omega-3 Fatty Acids are also polyunsaturated; they inhibit inflammation in the body. This type of fat is found in fatty fish, such as, salmon, sardines, whitefish, and herring. Flax seed oil, flax and hemp seeds, and walnuts are good sources of Omega 3's.

Cooking Oils have variable health benefits but are often chosen based on their cooking characteristics; these include olive oil; grape-seed oil; sesame, safflower, avocado and coconut oils. See below for a comparison.

Fruits: Are considered "red" only because of they often have too much sugar; people with diabetes or those who want to lose weight have to limit most fruits to two servings per day; some fruits such as berries may be considered as "free foods" because they are low in calories and have lots of vitamins. See below for a comparison of serving sizes.

Mushrooms: Are by nature somewhere between vegetables and animal meats in terms of their nutrient content. All mushrooms are rich in vitamins, minerals and even protein; they add a lot flavors to dishes when cooked. Avoid raw white button head mushrooms as when uncooked they contain unhealthy chemicals.

Beverages: Eliminate sodas and sugary drinks. Beers have carbs and should be consumed occasionally. Most wines and spirits are considered low in carbs but have to be consumed with caution because of their alcohol content.

Sugar & Sugar Substitutes: Cut back all types of sugars; if sugar substitutes are to be used, natural products such as stevia or agave extracts are preferred. They have no calories and as opposed to Sucralose (Splenda) they are not bad for the environment.

Sauces & Gravies; Condiments & Dressings: Use with discretion and pay attention to salt and preservative contents.

Herbs & Spices: Add calorie-free flavor and nutrients to foods and are considered "free foods" – use to taste.

Bars & Shakes: Pay attention to calories and ingredients; use when other natural foods are not readily available or when one has to increase protein intake (such as in vegetarian diets.) Whenever possible make your own shakes and add protein powder.

Supplements & Vitamins: Consult with your doctor or nutritionist.

Fast Foods, Pre-Made Meals (a.k.a. "TV dinners") and Concession Foods should be avoided.

NUTRITION LABELS

Reading Nutrition Labels

Nutrition labels provide useful information but may be confusing. Here are some key pointers about labels. The nutrition facts section of a food label shows the information on serving size, servings per container, total fat, saturated fat, cholesterol, sodium, total carbohydrate, dietary fiber, sugar, and protein.

- Serving size

Calories per serving correspond to the calories in the serving size as defined on the label. These are often listed as a certain number of pieces, ounces, or cups. Look at the serving size and be aware that you may need to do some calculations. For example, if you usually eat 2 cups of chili and a serving is defined as 1 cup, you will need to double the numbers to get the actual number of calories you are taking in.

- Carbohydrate Grams

Total carbohydrates on a label include sugars, complex (other) carbohydrates, and dietary fiber. Look at the grams of carbohydrate in the serving size. Usually if a food item provides 15 grams or more of carbohydrates per serving it is considered one serving of carbs. You should pay attention to the amount of sugar in the serving size. Since sugar is absorbed quickly, the more sugar in the serving size, the faster and higher blood glucose levels rise. Grams of sugar and fiber are counted as part of the total grams of total carbohydrate. If an item as has 5 grams or more fiber in a serving, subtract the fiber grams from the total grams of carbohydrate to yield the "net" carb. This is possible because fiber is not digested. Starches are molecules that are made of sugars linked together. Foods like potatoes, grains and legumes contain most of their calories as carbohydrate in starch form.

Sugars come in many chemical forms such as lactose, fructose, and sucrose, some sweeter than others. Lactose (milk sugar) is not sweet, but fructose (fruit sugar) is very sweet as is table or white sugar called sucrose. Sugar is rapidly absorbed into the blood stream. Some people who eat large amounts of sugar believe they feel a sugar "high" while others feel sick.

Fiber is a form of carbohydrate that is not broken down for energy. It provides no calories and does not affect blood sugar levels.

Sugar alcohols are neither "sugar" nor "alcohol" per se. They do provide fewer calories than sugar or starches and are used as sweeteners and bulking agents. Using sugar alcohol doesn't necessarily indicate that a food is low in carbohydrates. If eaten in excess, it may result in abdominal discomfort.

- Fat Grams

Fat is rich in calories; each gram of fat has nine calories. So a high-fat item is high in calories regardless of the type of fat in it. On a food label, total fat tells you how much fat is in a serving size. It is important to pay attention to the fat source. Good fats consist of mono and polyunsaturated fats, and bad fats include saturated and trans-fats. You also want to look at the grams of cholesterol. In a low-calorie diet that provides 1200 calories a day, the total fat intake is usually no more than 400 Calories (corresponding to 30% of total calories) or roughly 45 grams of fat. Paying attention to the fat content in food, you can avoid adding excess calories.

- Protein Grams

Look at the protein content per serving size. As a rule, one ounce of any meat source has 7 grams of protein. We suggest lean meat sources. In our meal plan, we recommend a total of 6 meals and snacks, each providing 15 to 30 grams of protein. So, in our meal plan a snack should contain 15 grams of protein or more. This could be 2 ounces of deli meat, a soy patty, low-fat cheese or a combination of almonds and cottage cheese. In general if the goal is to lose weight protein sources should not have more than 15 calories per gram of protein – ideally no more than 10. So a source of protein which has 10 grams of protein should not have more 150 calories (ideally 100.)

- Sodium

Pay attention to the sodium content. Ideally, try to aim to 3000 grams of sodium per day. There is a lot of hidden salt in foods. Watch out for canned foods, cheese, salad dressings, and packaged food. Try not to add table salt to food.

- Alcohol

What about alcohol? Alcohol provides more calories per gram than any other macronutrient type other than fat: 7 calories per gram. But, alcohol by itself is not a major culprit when it comes to weight gain. Remember your body has to destroy alcohol (in your liver), it cannot store it like fat or carbohydrates. So, calories from alcohol are not the same as those from food. However, alcoholic drinks often have additional calories from sugar (in the drink itself) or added juices for example. Some drinks even have fat calories such as cream. Avoid high sugar or mixed drinks.

> As a rule, for weight loss, avoid food items that have more than 10 calories per gram of protein; for example, if a protein bar has 15 grams of protein for a total of 300 calories (20 calories / gram of protein), that item is not suitable for weight loss.

MEAL CHALLENGES

Planning Ahead: Common Challenges with Meals

- Breakfast Challenges: Running Late

If you are a person who eats on the run, here are some suggestions for eating breakfast in the car, on the train, or at your work desk:

- Consider a protein shake that you make at home and bring in a commuter mug, with or without a protein bar (consult your health coach on good options for your eating plan).
- A container of sugar-free Greek-style yogurt with a piece of fruit is another alternative.
- If you are allowed to eat bread, pack a slice of whole grain bread or a few multi-grain flat breads and spread with light cream cheese or other low-fat alternatives: Two ounces of low-fat "Laughing Cow" and 6 – 8 high-fiber crackers.

Breakfast doesn't have to be your "normal traditional breakfast foods" such as cereal or pancakes. Some possible choices are leftovers (e.g. grilled chicken or shrimp with vegetables), chicken or a variety of soups, taco lettuce wraps, and turkey cold cuts with some fruit.

- Challenges at Lunch: Lack of time

Most people throughout the day do not have long breaks to de-stress or slowly eat a quiet lunch. In fact, the opposite is often the case. People whose lunch breaks are short (or just do not exist) have no choice but to eat a smaller (often cold) meal. For them, mid-morning and mid-afternoon snacks are very important and must serve as small meals to prevent hunger. For example, a yogurt with some cereal or a half of a sandwich would be a quick and easy choice. If lunch is poorly planned or skipped all together it will result in stress eating - triggered by hunger and lack of energy. This stress eating will result in grabbing handy pre-made and often fatty foods (e.g. pizza slices). If quick and easy healthy meals are eaten throughout the day, stress eating can be avoided.

- Business Lunches

Business lunches present a different challenge - social overeating. Here, lunch is not rushed because it is specifically scheduled for business conversation. However, it is difficult to eat just a salad at an hour long business lunch. In situations such as these, it is important that you remember to be mindful of your food choices. This involves watching portion sizes, side dishes, hidden calories, and desserts. Furthermore, do not feel tempted or pressured to eat foods because "you have to." Opt for sandwiches with protein, salads, and fruit. It is okay if you try new items - just be aware of how they are prepared. For example, a dish with a cream sauce is very high in calories, so that would not be a good option.

- Cafeteria Style Eating

Some people have to settle for cafeteria food, where the science of nutrition, healthy choices, and the art of cooking are rarely given priority. Now however, many cafeterias are offering salad bars, grilled foods, and healthier selections. Even though these selections may be more expensive than the fatty, deep fried, calorie-dense foods that are also available, they will provide you with a more nutritious and satisfying meal that is in line with your meal plan.

- Eating on the Road

Sales Reps, Commercial Drivers or people traveling long hours are often forced to eat lunches and dinners on the road. In most areas, food choices available on the road are not as much a problem as the time constraints and deadlines are for travelers. Even fast food outlets are beginning to offer reasonably healthy choices. However, if meeting the next client matters more than eating a healthy lunch, the end result is stress eating and weight gain. People who are traveling can bring along a cooler filled with healthy snacks, small meals, and water. Therefore, they are less likely to eat unhealthy foods because they are starving and pressed for time.

- Planning Dinners: Overeating

In our experience, majority of people eat a full dinner – unless they work the evening or night shifts. Going forward, you will learn to cook healthy dinners and save leftovers for future meals. The most challenging aspect regarding dinner is eating out. Plan on your choice of restaurants or take-out outlets. Look at menus on line before you pick a restaurant. If you are going out with friends, ask them to choose restaurants which offer menus you can select from. If your family members order food for you to pick up on your way home ask them to order items that are in line with your diet: lean protein choices with little or no fried foods or starches.

MEAL PLANNING: ORGANIZATIONAL SKILLS

Meal Planning: Plan to Be Organized and Pro-Active

To be able to cook a healthy meal at home you will need the following supplies:

- Food Scale
- Measuring Cup
- Small Snack Bags
- Saran Wrap
- Small Containers
- Tin Foil
- Cold Packs
- Cooler (for the car)
- Lunch Bags
- Low Cal Condiments
- Interesting spreads, seasoning and spices
- Frozen prepared meals
- Dry or canned soups

Planning is one of the most critical elements in a successful weight loss program. The best way to approach food shopping is to make a list in advance: a few minutes of pre-planning is remarkably effective in helping you meet your weight loss goals.

Keep a master shopping list, and if possible save it on your computer. Circle all items you need to buy each day or every time you go shopping. Remember, plan your shopping ahead and never go to the store hungry!

Examples of foods to keep in the house:

- Frozen meat & poultry
- Canned tuna in water
- Pre-portioned frozen fish steaks
- Low-fat cold cuts
- Soy foods such as veggie patties
- Broth and bouillon cubes
- Greek-style low or zero fat yogurt
- Low-fat cheeses
- Pre-cooked frozen shrimp
- A selection of herbal teas, diet sodas
- Sugar-free sweeteners (prefer natural)
- Frozen fruits & vegetables
- Sugar-free Jello, low-fat popcorn, healthy low-calories snacks
- Natural beef jerkies
- Nuts & seeds
- Variety of fresh fruits and vegetables
- Protein powder, shakes and bars

Finally clean up your kitchen pantries and refrigerators and throw out all items that are not in line with your program.

Summary

- If you have medical conditions, consult your doctor before beginning any meal plan.
- High protein meal plans are not suitable for people with kidney or liver failure.
- In case of food intolerance or allergies, look for replacements.
- You may personalize your meal plan with the help of a dietitian.
- Learn to choose foods wisely: Be mindful!
- Learn to cook simple dishes in batches.
- Eat slowly and frequently.
- Begin meals with proteins and fats, then carbohydrates.
- Avoid enriched starches, sweets and foods rich in saturated fats.
- Include foods rich in fiber in meals and snacks.

CALORIC ALLOWANCE

Daily Macronutrient Composition Guidelines Based on Caloric Allowance
- **Calorie range 1,000**
- Protein - 110 grams minimum • Carbs 75 grams or less
- Fat- 30 grams maximum • 1 fruit serving • 80 – 100 ounces water • Eat every 3 hours
- **Calorie range 1,200**
- Protein - 120 grams minimum • Carbs 75 grams or less • Fat - 40 grams maximum • 1 fruit serving • 80 - 100 ounces water • Eat every 3 hours
- **Calorie range 1,400**
- Protein - 120 grams minimum • Carbs 75 grams or less • Fat - 40 grams maximum • 1 - 2 fruit servings • 80 - 100 ounces water • Eat every 3 hours
- **Calorie range 1,600**
- Protein - 130 grams minimum • Carbs 75 grams or less • Fat - 45 grams maximum • 1 - 2 fruit servings • 80 - 100 ounces water • Eat every 3 hours
- **Calorie range 1,800**
- Protein - 140 grams minimum • Carbs 75 grams or less • Fat - 45

grams maximum • 1 - 2 fruit servings • 80 - 100 ounces water • Eat every 3 hours

PROTEIN SOURCES

Recommended Sources of Protein

- **Very Lean Sources of Protein (5 calories per gram of protein; 7 grams of protein per 1 oz cooked)**

Poultry: Chicken, Turkey, Cornish Hen (without skin, white meat only)
Fish: Cod, Flounder, Haddock, Halibut, Trout, Fresh or canned Tuna (canned in water and drained)
Shellfish: Clams, Crab, Lobster, Scallops, Shrimp
Dairy: Fat-free or 1 % Cottage Cheese (1/4 cup = 1 ounce), Fat-free Cheese, Plain Greek Yogurt
Eggs: Whites (2 whites = 1 ounce), Egg Substitute (1/4 cup = 1 ounce)

- **Lean Sources of Protein (10 calories per gram or protein; 7 grams of protein per 1 oz cooked)**

Beef: Round, Sirloin, Flank, Tenderloin, Roast (rib, chuck, rump), Ground Round
Pork: Lean Cuts of Ham, Canadian Bacon, Tenderloin, Center Loin Chop Lamb: Roast, Chop, Leg

Veal: Lean chop, Leg
Poultry: Dark Meat Chicken or Turkey (no skin), Duck
Fish: Catfish, Herring, Oysters, Salmon, Tuna (canned in oil, drained)
Dairy: Reduced fat Cheese such as Feta, Mozzarella and String cheese, Grated Parmesan (2 Tbs.)
Whole Egg: (limit for those with cholesterol problems)

- **Vegetarian Protein Sources (20-30 calories per gram of protein; 1 cup cooked per serving size)**

Beans: Black, White, Kidney, etc.: 15 grams of protein per cup cooked; 225-250 calories

Grains: Barley, Oats, Rice, Farro : Approx. 5-8 grams of protein per cup cooked; 160-200 calories

Legumes: Chickpeas, Edamame, Lentils: 15 grams per cup cooked; 190-270 calories

Soy Products: Light Tofu (Firm or Silken), Soy Burgers or Sausage; Seitan

Shakes: Rice Powder, Hemp Powder, Soy powder

FOOD COMPARISONS & SERVING SIZES

Nuts:

Nut	Almond	Cashew	Hazelnut	Peanut*	Pistachio	Walnut
Protein (gm) / oz	6	5	4	7	6	4
Numbers / oz	20	20	20	30	50	15 halves
Calories / oz	160	160	180	160	160	190

* a legume but often placed in the "nuts" category because it is consumed as dry nuts

Natural Nut Butters – About 2 grams of protein per 1 tbsp

Seeds:

Seed	Chia	Hemp	Pumpkin	Quinoa*	Sesame	Sunflower
Protein (gm) / oz	4	9	4	8	5	6
Tbsp / oz	2	3	2	1 Cup	3	4
Calories / oz	140	160	125	220	165	165

* measured as cooked; serving size of 1 cup

Comparison of Breads & Baked Goods:

Bread	White	Wheat	Rye	Hamburger Bun	Bagel	English Muffin	Wrap
Calories / 2 slices	220	220	320	200	300	120	200
Protein (gm)	8	10	12	6	10	4	6
Carbs (gm)	44	38	68	37	59	25	33

Comparison of Common Cooking Oils:

Oil	Olive	Coconut	Safflower	Canola	Grapeseed	Avocado
Calories / Tbsp	120	117	120	120	120	120
Smoke Point (degrees F)	374- 419	351	468	437	400	520
Oil Composition	73% Monosaturated	92% Saturated	77% Unsaturated	63% Monosaturated	71% Unsaturated	70% Monosaturated
Characteristics	Used for sautéing or salad dressings	Used for frying and baking	Flavorless & Versatile	Balanced	Versatile	Versatile but best for high temp cooking

Fermented Foods – Natural Probiotic Bacteria & Prebiotic Fiber:
    Kimchi: Pickled fermented cabbage, radish, eggplants., etc.
    Miso: Fungus fermented soybeans, barley rice and other grains
    Natto: High protein bacteria-fermented soybeans
    Tempeh: Fungus fermented soybeans
    Sauerkraut: Salt-pickled cabbage
    Kefir: Milk fermented by bacteria and yeast (no fiber)
    Kombucha: Fermented tea drink (no fiber)

Serving Size of Fruits:
    Apple -1 medium; Berries – 1/2 cup; Strawberries – 1 cup sliced; Cherries – 10 whole; Grapefruit – 1/2 of a whole; Grapes – 12; Mango – 1/2 whole; Melons – 1 cup cubed; Nectarine – 1 whole; Orange – 1 medium; Peach – 1 medium; Pear – 1 medium; Plum – 2 whole

A DAILY MEAL PLAN

A Simple Weekly Meal Plan:

This is an example of how to create a 1000 Calorie Low-Carb Low-Fat Dietary Plan:

Foods from different days may be interchanged or simply a one-day plan may be assembled with just preferred items;

For additional caloric allowance, portion sizes are increased accordingly.

There are many ways a dietary plan can be assembled. The key points are:

- Eat every 3 hours to keep the appetite hormones in check and to keep satiety signals up.
- Keep caloric intake down by cutting back on carbs and fats but not protein.
- Consume about 15 to 20 grams of protein with snacks and 30 to 40 grams of proteins with meals.
- Drink about 3 liters of water (including sugar-free, caffein-free and alcohol-free drinks.)
- Always track your intake.

- Monday

Breakfast 4 ounces 28 gm	4 egg white omelet with ¼ cup sliced mushrooms, ¼ cup diced onions, 1 Tbs grated parmesan cheese, and fresh or dried herbs to taste
Snack 1-2 ounces 7-14 gm	½ cup of 1% fat cottage cheese and ½ cup fresh blueberries
Lunch 5-6 ounces 35-42 gm	6 oz turkey breast and 2 cups garden salad with 2 Tbsp balsamic vinegar
Snack 1-2 ounces 7-14 gm	5 celery sticks with 12 almonds (½ oz)
Dinner 4-6 ounces 28-42 gm	5 oz grilled or roasted chicken breast, no skin; 1 ½ cups steamed green beans with ½ Tbs Smart Balance margarine
Snack	Optional

Calories: 940; Protein: 125 grams; Carbohydrate: 56 grams

NOTES:

- Tuesday

Breakfast 4 ounces 28 gm	1 cup 1% fat cottage cheese with ½ cup chopped bell peppers, seasoned with herbs as desired
Snack 1-2 ounces 7-14 gm	1 string cheese with 1 apple
Lunch 5-6 ounces 35-42 gm	5 oz of the grilled chicken from dinner and 2 cups tossed salad with 2 Tbsp balsamic vinegar
Snack 1-2 ounces 7-14 gm	2 oz smoked turkey breast with 5 fresh broccoli spears
Dinner 4-6 ounces 28-42 gm	4 oz grilled or roasted lean beef trimmed of fat (i.e., sirloin, tenderloin, or flank), 1 ½ cups steamed or grilled asparagus
Snack	Optional

Calories: 1040; Protein: 132 grams; Carbohydrates: 60 grams

NOTES:

- Wednesday

Breakfast 4 ounces 28 gm	4 oz smoked salmon, ½ medium tomato seasoned with black pepper to taste
Snack 1-2 ounces 7-14 gm	12 almonds with 5 celery sticks
Lunch 5-6 ounces 35-42 gm	5 oz left-over roast beef, 2 cups garden salad with 1 Tbsp low-calorie dressing
Snack 1-2 ounces 7-14 gm	¾ cup Greek yogurt with ½ cup raspberries
Dinner 4-6 ounces 28-42 gm	5 oz grilled tuna with 1 cup steamed zucchini with ½ Tbs Smart Balance margarine and 1 cup sweet red bell peppers, steamed or raw
Snack	Optional

Calories: 1000; Protein: 129 grams; Carbohydrate: 43 grams

NOTES:

- Thursday

Breakfast 4 ounces 28 gm	2 scrambled eggs with 2 oz Canadian bacon; 1 plum
Snack 1-2 ounces 7-14 gm	1 Lemon Razzy
Lunch 5-6 ounces 35-42 gm	6 oz canned tuna with 2 Tbsp light mayonnaise, ¼ cup chopped tomatoes, and ¼ cup chopped onion; 2 cups green salad
Snack 1-2 ounces 7-14 gm	1 string cheese with ½ medium yellow squash, sliced
Dinner 4-6 ounces 28-42 gm	6 oz grilled shrimp with 1 ½ cups steamed broccoli and 1 plum
Snack	Optional

Calories: 1020; Protein: 137 grams; Carbohydrates: 54 grams

NOTES:

- Friday

Breakfast 4 ounces 28 gm	4 egg white omelet with 1 cup chopped fresh spinach, 2 Tbs shredded light cheddar cheese, and herbs seasoned to taste
Snack 1-2 ounces 7-14 gm	15 walnut halves
Lunch 5-6 ounces 35-42 gm	5 oz chicken cut into strips and stir-fried with ½ cup onion, ½ cup red peppers, fresh garlic to taste. Try adding 2-3 Tbs sugar free salsa or some sliced fresh ginger root
Snack 1-2 ounces 7-14 gm	½ cup Greek yogurt with 1 pear
Dinner 4-6 ounces 28-42 gm	5 oz baked or broiled center cut pork chop with 1 cup asparagus and 1 large Portobello mushroom cap, both grilled; 1½ cups green salad with 2 Tbs balsamic vinegar
Snack	Optional

Calories: 1000; Protein: 113 grams; Carbohydrates: 67 grams

NOTES:

- Saturday

Breakfast 4 ounces 28 gm	1 soy burger with 2 Tbsp Feta cheese melted on top and ½ cup cherry tomatoes
Snack 1-2 ounces 7-14 gm	1 Lemon Razzy (a protein shake)
Lunch 5-6 ounces 35-42 gm	2 cups green salad with 6 oz extra lean ham, diced and mixed with 1 Tbs light mayonnaise
Snack 1-2 ounces 7-14 gm	2 oz smoked turkey breast with ½ grapefruit
Dinner 4-6 ounces 28-42 gm	5 oz grilled salmon with 1 cup well boiled cauliflower, mashed with 1 tsp Smart Balance and seasoned with salt and pepper; ½ medium cucumber peeled and sliced
Snack	Optional

Calories: 990; Protein: 116 grams; Carbohydrates: 47 grams

NOTES:

- Sunday

Breakfast 4 ounces 28 gm	4 egg white omelet with ¼ cup onion and 1 large Portobello mushroom cap, both diced, with 2 Tbsp Feta cheese and herbs seasoned to taste
Snack 1-2 ounces 7-14 gm	12 almonds and 5 celery sticks
Lunch 5-6 ounces 35-42 gm	6 oz shrimp stir-fried with 1 cup chopped red and green peppers, 1 cup summer squash, ½ cup chopped onion and fresh garlic to taste
Snack 1-2 ounces 7-14 gm	¾ cup Greek yogurt with ½ medium cucumber, peeled and sliced; 1 plum
Dinner 4-6 ounces 28-35 gm	5 oz grilled or roasted chicken breast, skinless; 1 cup steamed wax beans; 1½ cups tossed salad with 2 Tbs balsamic vinegar; 1 plum
Snack	Optional

Calories: 980; Protein: 114 grams; Carbohydrates: 73 grams

NOTES:

ADDITIONAL CHOICES: SIMPLE BREAKFASTS

- Scrambled egg whites and turkey sausage: 3 egg whites scrambled with 2 ounces of turkey sausage with 1 slice of low-carbohydrate wheat/whole grain bread.

(208 total calories, 7 grams fat, 10 grams carbohydrates, 28 grams protein)

- Omelet with spinach and feta: 1 whole egg plus 2 egg whites with 1/4 cup reduced fat crumbled feta cheese and 1/2 cup spinach (from last night's dinner), seasoned with fresh or dried herbs to taste. 1 slice of low-carbohydrate wheat/ whole grain bread, toasted.

(259 total calories, 9 grams fat, 14 grams carbohydrates, 27 grams protein)

- Cottage cheese and fresh strawberries: 1 cup of 1 % cottage cheese and 1/2 cup sliced strawberries.

(225 total calories, 4 grams fat, 22 grams carbohydrates, 25 grams protein)

- Western Omelet: 3 egg whites, 1/2 cup chopped peppers, 1/4 cup chopped onions and 1 ounce Monterey Jack cheese with 1 slice low-carbohydrate wheat/whole grain toast.

(233 total calories, 8 grams fat, 18 grams carbohydrates, 23 grams protein)

- Smoked Salmon Breakfast: 3 ounces smoked salmon and 1 Tbs. low-fat cream cheese spread on 2 slices low-carb toast

(275 total calories, 10 grams fat, 19 grams carbohydrates, 29 grams protein)

- Greek yogurt parfait: 1 cup (8 ounces) plain Greek yogurt blended with 1 cup frozen whole strawberries and 1 tablespoon milled flax seeds.

(210 total calories, 2.5 grams fat, 23 grams carbohydrates, 25 grams protein)

- Open-faced breakfast sandwich: 1 soy burger with 1 sunny-side-up egg on top and 1 slice low-carbohydrate wheat/ whole grain bread.

(240 total calories, 10 grams fat, 15 grams carbohydrates, 26 grams protein)

- Egg white and feta omelet: 4 egg whites with 1/4 cup reduced fat crumbled feta cheese seasoned with fresh or dried herbs to taste.

(134 total calories, 4.5 grams fat, 1 gram carbohydrates, 23 grams of protein)

- Asparagus and mushroom omelet: 1 whole egg and 3 egg

whites with 1/2 cup chopped asparagus and 1/4 cup chopped mushrooms.

(160 total calories, 5 grams fat, 7 grams carbohydrates, 22 grams protein)

- Western egg white omelet: 4 egg white omelet with 1/4 cup chopped bell peppers and 1/4 cup onions seasoned with 1 ounce of Monterey Jack cheese.

(179 total calories, 9 grams fat, 6 grams carbohydrates, 20 grams protein)

- Spinach and cheese egg white omelet: 4 egg whites with 1 cup chopped spinach and 1 ounce part skim mozzarella cheese.

(149 total calories, 4 grams fat, 3 grams carbohydrates, 26 grams protein)

- Egg white and feta omelet with bacon: 3 egg white omelet with 1/4 cup reduced fat crumbled feta cheese and 2 ounces of Canadian bacon.

(188 total calories, 6.5 grams fat, 2 grams carbohydrates, 30 grams protein)

- Scrambled egg whites and turkey sausage: 3 egg whites scrambled with 2 ounces of turkey sausage with 1 slice of low-carbohydrate wheat/whole grain bread.

(208 total calories, 7 grams fat, 10 grams carbohydrates, 28 grams protein)

- Smoked salmon with cheese: 3 ounces of smoked salmon with 1 ounce of Gouda cheese.

(250 total calories, 13 grams fat, 1 gram carbohydrates, 28 grams protein)

- Veggie Burger: 1 veggie burger with 1 fried egg on top and 1 slice low-carbohydrate wheat/whole grain bread.

(240 total calories, 10 grams fat, 15 grams carbohydrates, 24 grams protein)

- Cottage cheese: 1 cup 1% fat cottage cheese with 1/2 cup bell pepper strips.

(206 total calories, 4 grams fat, 16 grams carbohydrates, 24 grams protein)

- Cottage cheese and fresh blueberries: 1 cup 1% fat cottage cheese with 1/2 cup fresh blueberries.

(223 total calories, 4 grams fat, 30 grams carbohydrates 24 grams protein)

- Eggs and toast: 3 hard boiled eggs with 1 slice of low-carbohydrate whole grain bread.

(250 total calories, 15 grams fat, 9 grams carbohydrates, 24 grams protein)

- Grapefruit and cheese melt: 1/2 grapefruit with 1 slices of low-carbohydrate bread and 2 ounces of melted smoked gouda cheese.

(300 total calories, 16 grams fat, 23 grams carbohydrates, 18 grams protein)

- Greek yogurt smoothie: Blend 6 ounces of plain Greek yogurt with 1/2 cup blueberries (add water to develop consistency you like). Enjoy with 2 scrambled egg whites.

(165 total calories, 0 grams fat, 28 grams carbohydrates, 23 grams protein)

- Greek yogurt parfait: 6 ounces of plain Greek yogurt with 1/2 cup of raspberries and 12 almonds chopped on top.

(207 total calories, 8 grams fat, 18 grams carbohydrates, 19 grams protein)

ADDITIONAL CHOICES: SIMPLE LUNCHES

- Roast beef over salad greens: 4 ounces of roast beef over 2 cups salad greens and 2 Tbs. of your favorite low-calorie dressing.

(217 total calories, 6 grams fat, 14 grams carbohydrates, 29 grams protein)

- Turkey sandwich: 4 ounces oven-roasted turkey breast (left over from last night), 2 slices of low-carbohydrate wheat/whole grain bread with lettuce and tomato.

(227 total calories, 3 grams fat, 23 grams carbohydrates, 32 grams protein

- Grilled chicken over salad: 4 ounces of grilled chicken (left over from last night) with 1 oz crumbled goat cheese or feta over 2 cups salad greens and 2 tablespoons of your favorite low-calorie dressing.

(275 total calories, 9 grams fat, 18 grams carbohydrates, 33 grams protein)

- Ham wrap: 4 ounces low-sodium ham with lettuce and tomato with a low-carb/high-protein wrap (about 90 calories) dressed with mustard.

(222 total calories, 7 grams fat, 21 grams carbohydrates, 32 grams protein)

- Tuna salad: 4 ounces tuna (fresh or canned in water) with 1 Tbs. light mayonnaise on top of a large 2 cup garden salad with 2 Tbs. of your favorite low-calorie dressing, such as balsamic vinaigrette.

(240 total calories, 7 grams fat, 10 grams carbohydrates, 35 grams protein)

- Chef Salad: 1 ounce each of low sodium ham and turkey slices with 1 sliced hard-boiled egg over a large 2 cup garden salad with 2 tablespoons of your favorite low-calorie dressing, such as balsamic vinaigrette.

(218 total calories, 8 grams fat, 12 grams carbohydrates, 25 grams protein)

- Salmon over salad: 4 ounces salmon (left over from last night) over a large 2-cup garden salad with 2 Tbs. of your favorite low-calorie dressing, such as balsamic vinaigrette.

(238 total calories, 9 grams fat, 12 grams carbohydrates, 32 grams protein)

- Roast beef sandwich: 5 ounces of roast beef, 2 slices low-carbohydrate wheat/whole grain bread with lettuce and tomato. Enjoy with a garden salad and 2 Tbs. of your favorite low- calorie dressing, such as a balsamic vinaigrette.

(378 total calories, 7.5 grams fat, 32 grams carbohydrates, 45 grams protein)

- Turkey sandwich: 5 ounces oven-roasted turkey breast, 2 slices of low-carbohydrate wheat/whole grain bread with lettuce and tomato. Enjoy with a garden salad and 2 Tbs. of your favorite low-calorie dressing such as a balsamic vinaigrette.

(328 total calories, 3 grams fat, 24 grams carbohydrates, 41 grams protein)

- Tuna sandwich: 5 ounces canned tuna with 1 Tbs. light mayonnaise, 2 slices low-carbohydrate wheat/whole grain bread with lettuce and tomato.

(270 total calories, 7 grams fat, 22 grams carbohydrates, 37 grams protein)

- Ham sandwich: 4 ounces low-sodium ham, 2 slices low-carbohydrate wheat/whole grain bread with lettuce and tomato. Enjoy with a garden salad and 2 Tbs. of your favorite low-calorie dressing, such as a balsamic vinaigrette.

(268 total calories, 6 grams fat, 27 grams carbohydrates, 30 grams protein)

- Grilled chicken garden salad: 5 ounces of grilled chicken on top of a garden salad with 2 Tbs. of your favorite low-calorie dressing, such as a balsamic vinaigrette.

(248 total calories, 3.5 grams fat, 15 grams carbohydrates, 36 grams protein)

- Roast beef garden salad: 5 ounces of roast beef on top of a garden salad with 2 Tbs. of your favorite low-calorie dressing, such as a balsamic vinaigrette.

(296 total calories, 8 grams fat, 15 grams carbohydrates, 45 grams protein)

- Fresh tuna salad: 5 ounces canned tuna with 1 Tbs. light mayonnaise on top of a garden salad with 2 Tbs. of your favorite low-calorie dressing, such as a balsamic vinaigrette.

(266 total calories, 13 grams fat, 18 grams carbohydrates, 35 grams protein)

- Ham and turkey salad: 3 ounces of turkey and 2 ounces of low-sodium ham on top of a garden salad with 2 Tbs. of your favorite low-calorie dressing, such as a balsamic vinaigrette.

(286 total calories, 5 grams fat, 15 grams carbohydrates, 38 grams protein)

- Turkey salad: 4 ounces of oven-roasted turkey breast on top of a garden salad with 2 Tbs. of your favorite low-calorie dressing, such as a balsamic vinaigrette.

(256 total calories, 3 grams fat, 13 grams carbohydrates, 34 grams of protein)

- Grilled salmon salad: 4 ounces grilled salmon on top of a garden salad with 2 Tbs. of your favorite low-calorie dressing, such as a balsamic vinaigrette.

(238 total calories, 9 grams fat, 13 grams carbohydrates, 32 grams protein)

- Grilled sole with steamed broccoli and cauliflower: 4 ounces of grilled sole with 1/2 cup of steamed broccoli and 1/2 cup steamed cauliflower. Enjoy with a green salad and 2 Tbs. of your favorite low-calorie dressing, such as a balsamic vinaigrette.

(236 total calories, 2 grams fat, 18 grams carbohydrates, 37 grams protein)

- Grilled tenderloin with steamed spinach: 4 ounces of grilled or roasted tenderloin with 1/2 cup steamed spinach.

(275 total calories, 18 grams fat, 5 grams carbohydrates, 26 grams protein)

- Grilled turkey breast with steamed green beans and carrots: 4 ounces grilled or roasted skin-less turkey breast with 1 cup steamed green beans, 1/2 steamed carrots and a green salad with 2 Tbs. of your favorite low-calorie dressing, such as a balsamic vinaigrette.

(243 total calories, 3 grams fat, 25 grams carbohydrates, 32 grams protein)

- Grilled salmon with steamed cauliflower and collard greens: 5 ounces grilled salmon with 1/2 cup steamed cauliflower and 1 cup steamed collard greens.

(275 total calories, 12 grams fat, 12 grams carbohydrates, 24 grams protein)

ADDITIONAL CHOICES: SIMPLE DINNERS

- Roasted turkey and spinach: 5 ounces roasted skinless turkey over 2 cups wilted spinach, sautéed in non-stick pan with broth, seasoned with garlic and herbs and 1 Tbs. Promise Light margarine. Side salad with vinaigrette (optional).

(300 total calories, 7 grams fat, 20 grams carbohydrates, 43 grams protein)

- Grilled chicken with steamed green beans: 5 ounces of grilled or roasted skinless chicken breast with 2 cups steamed green beans and 1 Tbs. Smart Balance margarine. Side salad with vinaigrette (optional)

(325 total calories, 8 grams fat, 22 grams carbohydrates, 35 grams protein)

- Poached cod with steamed broccoli: 5 ounces of cod poached in broth with 2 cup steamed broccoli and 1 Tbs. Smart Balance margarine. Side salad with vinaigrette (optional)

(257 total calories, 7 grams fat, 14 grams carbohydrates, 39 grams protein)

- Sautéed shrimp and vegetables: 5 ounces shrimp sautéed with 1 cup summer squash or zucchini and 1/2 cup onion seasoned with herbs with 1 Tbs. Smart Balance margarine.

(244 total calories, 7 grams fat, 15 grams carbohydrates, 30 grams protein)

- Grilled chicken with portabella: 4 ounces grilled chicken breast, 2 grilled portabella mushroom caps and 1 ounce reduced fat feta cheese melted on top. Side salad with vinaigrette (optional).

(282 total calories, 7 grams fat, 23 grams carbohydrates, 34 grams protein)

- Broiled salmon with steamed asparagus: 5 ounces broiled salmon with 2 cups steamed aspara- gus drizzled with lemon and herbs. Side salad with vinaigrette (optional).

(340 total calories, 10 grams fat, 25 grams carbohydrates, 35 grams protein)

- Grilled sirloin steak with roasted cauliflower: 5 ounces of grilled sirloin served with 2 cups of oven-roasted cauliflower, seasoned with onion and garlic powder. Side salad with vinaigrette (optional).

(339 total calories, 13 grams fat, 21 carbohydrates, 37 grams protein)

- Grilled chicken with steamed green beans and 1/2 yam: 5 ounces of grilled or roasted skinless chicken breast with 1 cup steamed green beans. Enjoy with a 1/2 small yam sprinkled with cinnamon.

(296 total calories, 3 grams fat, 33 grams carbohydrates, 36 grams protein)

- Grilled sirloin steak with steamed asparagus and squash: 5 ounces of grilled or roasted sirloin with 1/2 cup of steamed asparagus and 1/2 cup steamed squash.

(285 total calories, 9 grams fat, 13 grams carbohydrates, 43 grams protein)

- Grilled tuna steak with steamed kale and roasted red peppers: 5 ounces grilled tuna with 1 cup steamed kale and 1/2 cup roasted red bell peppers. Enjoy with a green salad with 2 Tbs. of your favorite low- calorie dressing, such as reduced-calorie Italian.

(266 total calories, 4 grams fat, 21 grams carbohydrates, 40 grams protein)

- Grilled sole with steamed broccoli and cauliflower: 5 ounces of grilled sole with 1/2 cup of steamed broccoli and 1/2 cup steamed cauliflower. Enjoy with a green salad and 2 Tbs. of your favorite low-calorie dressing, such as a balsamic vinaigrette.

(287 total calories, 3 grams fat, 19 grams carbohydrates, 45 grams protein)

- Grilled tenderloin with steamed spinach: 4 ounces of grilled or roasted tenderloin with 1 cup steamed spinach. Enjoy with a green salad and 2 Tbs. of your favorite low-calorie dressing, such as a balsamic vinaigrette.

(340 total calories, 18 grams fat, 16 grams carbohydrates, 28 grams protein)

- Grilled turkey breast with steamed green beans and carrots: 4 ounces grilled or roasted skinless turkey breast with 1 cup steamed green beans, 1/2 cup carrots and a green salad with 2 table- spoons of your favorite low-calorie dressing, such as a balsamic vinaigrette.

(309 total calories, 4 grams fat, 30 grams carbohydrates, 27 grams protein)

- Grilled flank steak with steamed brussels sprouts and green beans: 4 ounces of grilled or roasted flank steak with 1/2 cup steamed broccoli and 1/2 cup steamed green beans. Enjoy with a green salad and 2 Tbs. of your favorite low-calorie dressing, such as a reduced-calorie Italian.

(375 total calories, 12 grams fat, 23 grams carbohydrates, 40 grams protein)

- Grilled salmon with steamed cauliflower and collard greens: 5 ounces grilled salmon with 1/2 cup steamed cauliflower and 1 cup steamed collard greens.

(277 total calories, 12 grams fat, 12 grams carbohydrates, 33 grams protein)

- Grilled chicken with steamed snow peas and portabella mushroom: 4 ounces grilled or roasted skinless chicken breast with 1/2 cup steamed snow peas and 1 grilled portabella mushroom cap. Enjoy with a green salad and 2 Tbs. of your favorite low-calorie dressing, such as a balsamic vinaigrette.

(250 total calories, 4 grams fat, 15 grams carbohydrates, 36 grams protein)

- Tuna salad: 4 ounces tuna (canned in water) with 1 Tbs. light mayonnaise on top of a garden salad with 2 Tbs. of your favorite low-calorie dressing, such as a balsamic vinaigrette.

(273 total calories, 9 grams fat, 17 grams carbohydrates, 36 grams protein)

- Grilled salmon salad: 4 ounces grilled salmon on top of a garden salad with 2 Tbs. of your favorite low-calorie dressing, such as a balsamic vinaigrette.

(238 total calories, 9 grams fat, 13 grams carbohydrates, 32 grams protein)

- Chef salad: 2 ounces of oven-roasted turkey breast, 2 ounces of low-sodium ham and 1 ounce of low-fat American cheese on top of a garden salad with 2 Tbs. of your favorite low-calorie dressing.

(325 total calories, 9 grams fat, 17 grams carbohydrates, 38 grams protein)

- Grilled halibut with squash and green beans: 5 ounces of grilled halibut with 1/2 cup steamed squash and 1/2 cup steamed green beans. Enjoy with a green salad and 2 Tbs. of your favorite low-calorie dressing, such as a balsamic vinaigrette.

(300 total calories, 5 grams fat, 25 grams carbohydrates, 40 grams protein)

- Grilled cod with broccoli and carrots: 5 ounces of grilled cod with 1/2 cup steamed broccoli and 1/2 cup steamed carrots. Enjoy with a green salad and 2 Tbs. of your favorite low-calorie dressing, such as a balsamic vinaigrette.

(359 total calories, 3 grams fat, 17 grams carbohydrates, 40 grams protein)

ADDITIONAL CHOICES: EASY SNACKS

- Cottage cheese with blueberries: 1/2 cup of 1% fat cottage cheese and 1/2 cup of blueberries mixed in.

(122 total calories, 1 gram fat, 15 grams carbohydrates, 15 grams protein)

- Almonds and cucumber: 12 almonds and 1 cup of cucumber slices dipped in low-fat tzatziki sauce.

(145 total calories, 9 grams fat, 4 grams carbohydrates, 5 grams protein)

- Greek yogurt with raspberries: 6 ounces of plain Greek yogurt with 1/2 cup of raspberries.

(142 total calories, 0.5 grams fat, 18 grams carbohydrates, 18 grams protein)

- Ham lettuce wrappers with bell peppers: 2 ounces of low-sodium ham wrapped in romaine lettuce leaves (dipped in mustard) with 1/2 cup sliced bell peppers.

(113 total calories, 3 grams fat, 8 grams carbohydrates, 13 grams protein)

- Pistachios and celery sticks: 25 pistachios and 8 medium celery sticks.

(110 total calories, 6.5 grams fat, 11 grams carbohydrates, 4 grams protein)

- Protein snack bar: 1 protein snack bar, such as Weight Wise or Luna (150 calorie range with 15 grams protein).

(150 total calories, 5 grams fat, 15 grams carbohydrates, 15 grams protein)

- Greek yogurt and blueberries: 6 ounces plain Greek yogurt and 1/2 cup blueberries.

(163 total calories, 0 grams fat, 28 grams carbohydrates, 17 grams protein)

- Celery dippers with cheese: 1 low-fat cheese stick and 8 celery stalks dipped in 2 tablespoons low-fat tzatziki sauce.

(146 total calories, 6 grams fat, 12 grams carbohydrates, 12 grams protein)

- Cottage cheese with blueberries: 1/2 cup of 1 % cottage cheese with 1/2 cup blueberries.

(122 total calories, 1 gram fat, 15 grams carbohydrates, 15 grams protein)

- Turkey roll-ups with bell peppers: 2 ounces low-sodium turkey rolled up in lettuce leaves dipped in mustard with 1/2 cup sliced peppers.

(120 total calories, 1.5 grams fat, 9 grams carbohydrates, 13 grams protein)

- Protein bar: Protein snack bar such as Weight Wise or Luna (150 calorie range with 15 grams protein).

(150 total calories, 5 grams fat, 15 grams carbohydrates, 15 grams protein)

- Almonds with broccoli spears: 12 almonds with 1 cup broccoli spears dipped in 2 tablespoons low-fat dressing.

(140 total calories, 8 grams fat, 8 grams carbohydrates, 9 grams protein)

- Pistachios with plums: 25 pistachios and 2 plums.

(145 total calories, 7 grams fat, 20 grams carbohydrates, 4 grams protein)

- Tomato and feta: 1 large, sliced tomato with 1/4 cup reduced fat crumbled feta.

(103 total calories, 5 grams fat, 8 grams carbohydrates, 9 grams protein)

- Cottage cheese and berries: 1/2 cup of 1% fat cottage cheese and 1/2 cup of blueberries mixed in. (122 total calories, 1 grams fat, 15 grams carbohydrates, 15 grams of protein)

- Almonds and celery sticks: 12 almonds and 15 celery sticks.

(115 total calories, 7.5 grams fat, 11 grams carbohydrates, 3 grams protein)

- Walnuts and cucumber sticks: 15 walnut halves and 1/2 cup of cucumber sticks.

(185 total calories, 16 grams fat, 5 grams carbohydrates, 4 grams of protein)

- Turkey lettuce wraps with bell peppers: 2 ounces of smoked turkey breast wrapped in romaine lettuce leaves with 1/2 cup bell peppers.

(120 total calories, 1.5 grams fat, 9 grams carbohydrates, 14 grams of protein)

Ham lettuce wraps with bell peppers: 2 ounces of low-sodium ham wrapped in romaine lettuce leaves with 1/2 cup bell peppers.

(113 total calories, 3 grams fat, 8 grams carbohydrates, 13 grams protein)

- Protein Bar: 1 low-carbohydrate protein bar.

(150 total calories, 5 grams fat, 15 grams carbohydrates, 15 grams of protein)

- Cheese sticks: 2 part-skim mozzarella cheese sticks.

(160 total calories, 12 grams fat, 2 grams carbohydrates, 14 grams of protein)

- Cottage cheese

and pear: 1/2 cup of 1% fat cottage cheese and 1 pear.

(186 total calories, 1 gram fat, 30 grams carbohydrates, 14 grams protein)

- Greek yogurt parfait: 6 ounces of plain Greek yogurt with 1/2 cup of raspberries.

(122 total calories, 0 grams fat, 15 grams carbohydrates, 16 grams protein)

- Greek yogurt with agave nectar: 6 ounces of plain Greek yogurt with 1 Tbs. of agave nectar mixed in.

(150 total calories, 0 grams fat, 23 grams carbohydrates, 15 grams protein)

RECIPES: EGGS

Tex-Mex Egg White Scramble with Cheese

Ingredients

½ cup	Pure (liquid) Egg White
2 tbsp	Salsa - mild (red or green)
1 tbsp	Olive oil
1 oz	Feta or other white cheese
1 tsp	Salt
1 tsp	Dry oregano

Instructions

A quick healthy meal for one person – often a breakfast – is to scramble egg whites in salsa with cheese. We recommend organic egg whites usually purchased in small cartons.

1. Heat olive oil over medium heat in a small non-stick pan.
2. Spread 1 tbs of oil to cover the surface of the pan – may dispose of excess oil.
3. Add salsa and then quickly the egg white. Turn temperature to low medium.
4. Add pieces of cheese and seasoning (here just salt and oregano but may add your preferred mix of herbs).

5. Cook for 2-3 minutes then using a wooden spoon gently mix the egg until scrambled firm but not dry (5 minutes total).

You can add a side of avocado or tomato slices.

You may choose to eat crackers, or a slice of bread toasted dry with this recipe (calories not included).

Nutrition Facts: Total protein about 30 g; total calories estimated at 200 calories from suggested sides or crackers are not included.

Callaloo with Smoked Fish and Scrambled Eggs

Ingredients

10 oz or 1 large fillet	Smoked trout or white fish
4 large	Eggs
½ tsp	Black pepper
¼ tsp	Salt
3	Fresh chives, chopped
2 tbsp	Olive oil
3 tbsp	Plain yogurt
4 cups	Callaloo, chopped
1 medium	Onion, chopped

Instructions

1. Sauté chopped onion and callaloo with 1 tbsp of olive oil in a skillet.
2. May add ½ cup of water or vegetable broth for moisture.
3. Cover and cook at low temperature.
4. Stir every 5 minutes.
5. Separate the flesh from the bones and skin of the fish and break into flakes.
6. Using a whisk, beat the eggs in a bowl with the salt, pepper, and chives.
7. In a small pan heat oil and cook egg mixture at low heat mixing continuously until eggs are scrambled but still runny. Set aside.
8. Add fish flakes to callaloo, mix well.
9. Now add eggs and yogurt and mix well.
10. Serve immediately.

May replace callaloo with spinach.
May eat with crackers or in low carb wrap.

Nutrition Analysis:
Estimated per serving: Calories 200; Protein 24 grams.

Creamy Eggs with Smoked Fish

Ingredients

1   Large smoked trout or white fish (about 10 ounces)
4   Large eggs
1/4 tsp Salt
1/4 tsp Freshly ground black pepper
3 tbsp Chopped fresh chives
4   Slices whole wheat bread (about 4 ounces total)
1 tbsp Good olive oil
3 tbsp Non-fat, plain yogurt

Instructions

The combination of smoked fish and scrambled eggs—whether served for breakfast, brunch, or as a light dinner—is a great favorite at my house. You can find smoked fish at many supermarkets and delicatessens now. I like to serve the eggs and fish on crunchy toast made from whole wheat, whole grain, or even country-style bread. The eggs are stirred while they cook with a whisk to ensure that the curds are small. Conventionally they are finished with cream, but yogurt gives them a little acidity and creaminess and stops the cooking. The eggs could also be served with sautéed fresh tomatoes, mushrooms or spooned over salad greens lightly seasoned with olive oil and white wine vinegar.

1. Separate the flesh from the bones and skin of the fish, and break each fillet into pieces or flakes, following the natural lines of the fish.
2. Using a whisk, beat the eggs in a bowl with the salt, pepper, and chives.
3. At serving time, toast the bread. Place one piece of toast on each of 4 plates and arrange the fish around the toast.
4. Heat the oil in a sturdy skillet or saucepan.
5. When it is hot, add the egg mixture.
6. Cook over medium to low heat, mixing continuously with a whisk to create the smallest possible curds.

7. Continue cooking for about 2 minutes, until the mixture is creamy, but still slightly runny.
8. Remove the pan from the heat, and add the yogurt. Mix well.
9. The mixture should be moist and soft. Spoon onto the toasts, dividing the eggs among the 4 plates. Serve immediately.

As part of your meal plan, this recipe can be used as meal, or as a snack. The added salt is optional.

Nutrition Analysis (per serving size of 166 g):

Calories 320; Fat 15 g; Cholesterol 270 mg; Carbohydrates 15 g; Protein 29 g.

Adapted from It Must Be My Metabolism by Reza Yavari, MD (recipe by Jacques Pepin)

Huevos Rancheros Blanco

Ingredients

1 small carton Egg White (prefer organic) about 30 tbsp (2 cups)
1 can   Organic Black Beans, drained and rinsed
4 oz   Cheese, white low fat (such as Oaxaca part skim string cheese), chopped
1   Poblano, seeds and ribs removed, chopped
1 large or 2 small Jalapeno, seeds and ribs removed, chopped
4 tbsp (generous) Salsa
1 bunch   Cilantro, chopped
8   Corn Tortillas, heated on a non-stick pan until slightly brown on one side
1 tbsp   Olive oil
2 tsp   Coriander Powder
2 tsp   Salt

Instructions

1. Heat two tbsp of olive oil then add chopped Poblano pepper and jalapeno.
2. Sauté till slightly browned or about 10 minutes - stir every 2-3 minutes.
3. Add salsa, mix then add beans.
4. Cook at medium heat for 5 minutes then pour in liquid egg white, coriander powder and cook for another 5 minutes mixing well to evenly scrambled.
5. Add salt to taste.
6. Visually divide pan content in 4 quarters.
7. Distribute each quarter onto 2 tortillas then add cheese and cilantro.
8. Serve and save remainder in the refrigerator for later meals.

Each serving (of two tacos) could be eaten from a bowl skipping calories from 2 tortillas (110 calories.)

Nutrition Analysis:

Estimated for two tacos: Calories 280; Protein 28 grams.

Mexican Frittata with Sausage

Ingredients

1 carton (20 servings)   Egg Whites

4 Eggs Whole

4 Chicken Sausage Links

½ package (5 oz)   Oaxaca Part Skim Cheese, sliced into "ribbons"

1 Large onion, chopped

2 Poblano Peppers, chopped

2 Jalapeno Peppers, chopped

4 Tomatillos, sliced

2 tbsp Oregano

2 tbsp Chili Powder

2 tbsp Paprika (smoked preferred)

2 tsp Salt

½ tsp Annotto / Anchiote oil (optional)

4 tbsp Olive Oil

Cilantro – chopped for garnish

Instructions

1. Pre-heat oven to 350°.
2. Sauté chopped onion, peppers, tomatillo and sausage slices in 2 tbsp of olive oil for about 10 minutes or till links are browned – let cool to room temperature.
3. In a big bowl mix whole eggs, liquid egg white, seasoning (and anchiote oil for color – if desired).
4. Heat 2 tbsp of olive oil in a platter in the oven.
5. Add sautéed veggies and sausage with cheese ribbons to the egg mixture and pour in platter.
6. Bake at 350° for 15 to 20 minutes.
7. Garnish with chopped cilantro.

Nutrition Analysis:

Estimated per serving size: Calories 220; Protein 27 grams.

This recipe contains 24 egg whites, sausage and cheese adding to about 220 grams of protein. A serving size of 1/8th of the platter has about 27 grams of protein for only about 220 calories. The frittata can be divided into 8 serving sizes and frozen in plastic wrap or containers for future. Chicken sausage may be replaced with soy links for a vegetarian alternative.

Scrambled Egg Tacos

Ingredients

- 6   Egg Whites
- 2   Whole Eggs
- 2 ounces or ¼ of package   String Cheese – Prefer Oaxaca part skim
- 2   Jalapeno, sliced and roasted in advance in the oven or on a dry pan
- 2   Pickled oed onion, sliced and marinated in lemon juice overnight
- 1 tbsp Olive oil
- 1 tsp Salt
- 4   Corn tortilla

Cilantro – chopped for garnish

Instructions

1. Heat olive oil in a non-stick pan at medium temperature.
2. Add eggs and cheese and mix while heating.
3. Briefly heat the corn tortillas.
4. Add 1/4 of scrambled eggs to each tortilla.
5. Place one or two slices of roasted jalapeno in each taco.
6. Garnish with pickled onion and chopped cilantro.
7. Add additional salt and chili powder or salsa to taste.

This recipe has 8 egg whites and two ounces of string cheese for a total of about 55 grams of protein. Each taco therefore contains about 14 grams of protein. Serving size is therefore 2 tacos containing about 30 grams of protein and only about 445 calories (of which about half are from the tortillas.) Could cook the eggs in advance and freeze portions for future.

Nutrition Analysis:

Serving size of 2 tacos: Calories 445; Protein 30 grams.

RECIPES: CHICKEN

Sofrito Chicken with String Beans

Ingredients

- 2 lbs — Chicken breast – boneless, skinless
- 1 cup — Chicken or vegetable broth
- 1 bag or 12 oz — String beans – prefer thin French beans
- ½ cup — Lemon Juice
- 2 medium — Onion, chopped
- 2 cloves — Garlic, minced
- 1 bunch — Scallion, thinly chopped (optional)
- ½ batch — Parsley or Cilantro – for garnish

Sofrito

2 tbsp	Olive oil
4	Green Peppers, seeds and ribs removed
2	Red Bell peppers, seeds and ribs removed
2 large	Tomatoes, cut
2 medium	Onions, chopped
2 cloves	Garlic, chopped
1 batch	Cilantro, chopped

Instructions

1. Add all sofrito ingredients together in a blender to puree
2. Pour into small containers and keep extra sofrito frozen until ready to use.
3. In a large skillet heat 4 tbsp of olive oil.
4. Add 4 tbsp of sofrito.
5. Cook at medium temperature for 4 minutes till sofrito is fragrant.
6. Add garlic, onions and string beans (cut 1" long) and cook for 5 minutes.
7. Add boneless skinless chicken breast strips or 1" cut pieces and sauté for 5 minutes or until slightly browned.
8. Now add broth and lemon juice, oregano (or an herb mixture such as *herbs de France*) cook for an additional 8 minutes.
9. Finish by adding garnish such as parsley or cilantro and chopped scallions on top.

Nutrition Analysis:
Estimated for one serving size (4 oz): Calories 280; Protein 43 grams.

Pollo Guisado with Finger Potatoes

Ingredients

2-3 lbs	Chicken thighs – boneless skinless
2 tbsp	Adobo blend seasoning
8 oz	Tomato sauce
2 tbsp	Olive oil
½ cup	Sofrito (see recipe in the Sides section)
1 cup	Chicken broth
¼ cup	Pimento-stuffed Spanish olives
1 tsp	Ground cumin
1	Bay leaf
½ tsp	Annotto / Anchiote oil (optional)
1 tsp	Coriander seed
12	Fingerling potatoes, washed but not peeled

Cilantro - chopped for garnish

Instructions

1. Season chicken with Adobo and brown in olive oil in a heavy pot at medium temperature 5 minutes on each side.

2. Add the other ingredients and cook for 35 minutes stirring every 10 minutes.

3. Bring two quarts of water to a boil.

4. Gently add fingerling potatoes and boil till fork tender – about 30 minutes.

5. Add salt, pepper and chili powder to taste.

Nutrition Analysis:

Estimated per serving size of 2 chicken thighs and 3 potatoes: Calories 716; Protein 63 grams.

Grilled chicken with Warm Black Bean Salsa

Ingredients

2 lbs	Boneless, Skinless Chicken Breasts – thin cuts (or 150 grams per breast)
2 tbsp	Olive oil

Dry Spice Mix

2 tbsp	Ground Cumin
1 tbsp	Chili Powder
2 tbsp	Oregano
2 tbsp	Coriander Powder
2 tsp	Salt

Black Bean Salsa

2 large	Poblano Peppers
2	Jalapeno Peppers
1 large or 2 mediums	Red Onion, chopped into small squares
2 cloves	Fresh Garlic, minced
1 can	Organic Cooked Black Beans, drained and rinsed
1 can	Organic Diced Tomato
2 tsp	Cumin Seeds (crushed) or Powder
2 tsp	Salt, may adjust to taste later
2	Juice of 2 Limes

Fresh Cilantro chopped

2 tbsp	Olive oil
1 cup	Vegetable Broth

Instructions

1. Put chicken breast in big bowl add oil then turn over breasts several time each time adding spice mix. All breasts should be covered by oil and spice mix. Set aside.

2. Cut peppers in halves lengthwise, remove seeds, roast in oven at high temperature (450 +) for about 10 minutes or until skin browned.

3. Peel and chop (remove skin in cold water – optional)

4. In a non-stick pan heat olive oil then add chopped onion, peppers and garlic.

5. Cook at medium temperature until onions are slightly translucent – do not brown.

6. Add diced tomatoes, mix. Add black beans and mix.

7. Simmer in 1 cup of vegetable broth (about 15 min) or until tomato pieces and beans are soft.

8. Adjust salt. Add lime juice and garnish with cilantro. Serve warm.

9. In a grill pan fry 6 chicken breasts 2 minutes on each side at medium temperature.

10. May add dry white wine in the last minute.

Serve chicken breast with 3 tablespoons of warm salsa on the side or on top. Add sautéed spinach or Swiss chard as a side vegetable if you wish. May also save salsa for tostadas and tacos.

Nutrition Analysis: Estimated per serving: Calories 375; Protein 37 grams.

Eggplant Split Pea Stew with Chicken

Ingredients

2 to 2.5 lbs	Chicken Thighs boneless skinless –

3 medium size or about 3 lbs Eggplants, washed and sliced then cut into 1-inch cubes

1 cup	Split Peas, washed
4 medium	Onion, cut in halves and sliced ½ inch wide
2 cups	Vegetable Broth
4 tbsp	Tomato Paste
3 tbsp	Olive oil
1 tbsp	Paprika
1 tbsp	All Spice – (may choose another blend)
1 tbsp	Ancho or Guajillo Chili powder

Instructions

1. First prepare eggplants:

2. In a large oven-resistant platter or tray gradually mix eggplant chunks with 2 tbsp of olive oil – may use a spray.

3. Then add your preferred All Spice mix evenly to all eggplant chunks.

4. Place the container in a preheated oven and roast at 400° for about 20 minutes turning eggplant pieces once so they brown on both sides.

5. Meanwhile in a large pot or Dutch oven, sauté onions in 1 tbsp of oil for 5 minutes, then add chicken thighs.

6. Add paprika and brown chicken for about 15 minutes.

7. Add broth, split peas, tomato paste, chili powder and mix well.

8. Bring to a boil and cook at medium temperature for about 20 minutes.

9. Add eggplant chunks and mix well.

10. Simmer for another 10 minutes.

11. Salt to taste.

This stew may be reheated several times and eventually frozen in small container for future meals. It is very satisfying with no starch, but you may wish to have a serving of rice or noodles with it (add extra calories.)

Nutrition Analysis (8 servings):
Estimated per serving: Calories 350; Protein 35 grams.

Cuban Black Bean (Caraotas Negras) with Chicken Sausage

Ingredients

1 can	Organic Black Beans, drained and rinsed
5	Chicken Links sausage, cut in 1 cm pieces
1	Bell Pepper, chopped
1	Poblano Pepper, chopped
1	Jalapeño Pepper, chopped
2 medium	Onions, chopped
2 cloves	Garlic, chopped and crushed
1 cup	Vegetable or Chicken Broth
1 tbsp	White Vinegar
1 tbsp	Olive Oil
2 tbsp	Cumin Ground
1 tbsp	Cinnamon
2 tbsp	Coriander Powder

Instructions

1. Heat olive oil in a non-stick pan.

2. Mix chopped onion, peppers and sausage links and cook at medium temperature until onion is soft and sausage is slightly browned.

3. Add black beans and spices, mix.

4. Pour in broth, add white vinegar and cook at low temperature for 15 to 20 minutes. Salt to taste.

Nutrition Analysis:

Estimated per serving: Calories 340; Protein 30 grams.

Chinese Creole Chicken

Ingredients

4 lbs   Chicken Breast Skinless Boneless

May use chicken strips or tenders

Marinade:

½ cup   Soy Sauce

½ cup   Lemon Juice

2 tbsp   Sesame oil – prefer toasted

2 tbsp   Honey

2 tbsp   Chili Sauce – prefer Sriracha

2 tbsp   Ginger fresh grated

2 tbsp   Creole herb mixture

1 tbsp   Olive oil

Instructions

1. Mix ingredients to make marinade.

2. Soak chicken tenders in marinade for 30 minutes while heating oven to 400°.

3. Take chicken out of the marinade, add the Creole mixture to both sides of chicken strips.

4. Heat olive oil in an oven-resistant or a skillet a for a few minutes.

5. Place chicken in the container and cook in oven for 30 min; flip chicken strips and broil for 5 to 8 minutes.

Nutrition Analysis:

Estimated per serving: Calories 230; Protein 42 grams.

Chicken with Vinegar Sauce

Ingredients

6 skinless chicken legs (about 2 3/4 pounds)

Seasoning mixture

1 tsp Dried oregano

1 tsp Dried marjoram

3/4 tsp Salt

1/2 tsp Freshly ground black pepper

1/2 tsp Good olive oil

1/4 cup Balsamic vinegar

1/4 cup Dry red wine

1/2 cup Trimmed and minced scallions

2 tbsp Catsup

1/2 cup Homemade chicken stock or low-salt canned chicken broth

4 tbsp Peeled and thinly sliced garlic

Instructions

This is a classic chicken dish from my home region of France, but I use skinless chicken legs to make the recipe less caloric. Notice that the acidity of the vinegar and wine reduction goes especially well with the chicken. If you have any leftovers, pick the meat off the bones, mix it with any remaining sauce, and serve as a type of ragout over pasta. You can also stuff an omelet with the leftover mixture, and serve it with a green salad for a hearty meal.

Combine the seasoning mixture ingredients in a small bowl.

1. Brush a large heavy saucepan or nonstick skillet with the olive oil, and heat it until hot.

2. Add the chicken legs in one layer, and sprinkle the seasoning mix over them.

3. Cook the legs, covered, over medium to low heat for 10 minutes.

4. Turn the legs over, cover again, and cook them for 10 minutes on the other side. The chicken should be well browned on all sides. Using tongs, transfer the legs to a serving platter, and set them aside in a warm place while you prepare the sauce.

5. Add the vinegar and red wine to the crystallized juices in the saucepan, bring the mixture to a boil, stirring, and boil it for 30 seconds.

6. Then add the scallions, catsup, chicken stock, and garlic.

7. Boil for about 2 minutes, until the mixture is reduced to about 1 cup of concentrated liquid.

8. To serve, discard any juices that have collected around the chicken on the platter, and drizzle the sauce over the legs. Serve.

Nutrition Analysis (per serving size of 264 g): Calories 290; Fat 9 g; Cholesterol 175 mg; Carbohydrates 6 g; Protein 42 g.

Adapted from It Must Be My Metabolism by Reza Yavari, MD (recipe by Jacques Pepin)

Chicken Pinchos with Black Beans

Ingredients

2 lbs	Chicken Thighs, boneless cut into 1-inch cubes
2 tbsp	Adobo seasoning blend
1 cup	Lemon juice
4 tbsp	Olive oil
2 packs	Sazon (if homemade 2 tbsp)
2 cans	Organic Black Beans
4 tbsp	Salsa, mild
8	Wooden skewers

Instructions

A **pincho** is a small snack, typically eaten in bars, traditional in northern Spain. They are called *pinchos* because many of them have a *pincho* (Spanish for *spike*), typically a toothpick or skewer.

1. Prep the chicken:
2. Soak chicken cubes in lemon juice in a big bowl for 5 to 10 minutes.
3. Then drain all the lemon juice.
4. Add olive oil, blend well so all pieces are covered.
5. Add Adobo mix and toss well then add Sazon (prefer homemade Sazon blend or at least make sure there is no MSG in the commercial product) and toss.
6. Cover and refrigerate for about 2 hours.
7. If using wood skewers soak them in water for about 2 hours or longer
8. Now prepare the black beans:
9. It is best to use dry beans but you need to soak them overnight and boil them for a few hours. Organic canned black beans are an acceptable alternative.
10. Drain beans in a colander.
11. Bring water to a boil, add beans and boil at medium temperature for about 30 minutes or until soft inside (make sure there is always plenty of water in the pot while boiling)
12. Carefully pour out hot water thru the colander and set beans aside to cool.
13. Take about one third of beans and put in a blender with mild salsa and pulse a few times.

14. Add blender mixture with beans to a bowl stir and refrigerate.

15. When ready to grill pinchos take beans out and bring to room temperature.

16. May add a few drops of balsamic vinegar before serving and salt to taste.

17. Place chicken on 8 skewers and cover chicken with additional olive oil and add seasoning as needed.

18. Place skewers in a row on a grill tray if broiling or directly on a grill top.

19. Grill or broil at high temperature for about 5 minutes on either side.

20. May add more oil to keep moist (no worries because extra oil drips into the bottom tray when broiling or burns off in the grill).

21. Cut one cube to make sure it is cooked right if not, cook for another 5 minutes.

22. Serve with a side of black beans and garnish with chopped cilantro.

Nutrition Analysis: Estimated per serving (about 4 oz of chicken): Calories 240; Protein 33 grams. Could eat more chicken if 4 oz is not enough.

Chicken in Red Wine Sauce

Ingredients

1 1/2 tbsp Good olive oil

12   Small pearl onions, peeled

1/2 tsp Sugar

8   Medium mushrooms, quartered

1/2 cup Finely chopped onion

1 tbsp Finely chopped garlic

1   Sprig fresh thyme

1   Bay leaf

1 1/2 cups Robust, fruity red wine

4   Boneless, skinless chicken breasts

2 tsp Dark soy sauce

3/4 tsp Freshly ground black pepper

1 tsp Potato starch dissolved in 2 tablespoon water

Instructions

This is a simple but elegant way to prepare chicken with a minimum amount of calories and a maximum amount of flavor.

1. Heat 1 tablespoon of the oil in a skillet, and add the pearl onions, sugar, mushrooms, and 1/2 cup water.

2. Bring to a boil, cover, and boil for 3 to 4 minutes.

3. Remove the cover and keep cooking over high heat until the water has evaporated.

4. Continue cooking until the onions and mushrooms take on a dark brown color.

5. Remove the mushrooms and onions from the skillet and set them aside in a bowl.

6. Add the chopped onion, garlic, thyme, bay leaf, and wine to the skillet.

7. Place the chicken breasts in the wine mixture in the skillet so they do not overlap and bring to a boil.

8. Reduce the heat, and simmer very gently for 7 to 8 minutes.

9. Add the soy sauce, pepper, and dissolved potato starch, and mix well.

10. Return the mushrooms and onions to the stew in the skillet, heat gently for 1 minute, and serve.

As part of your meal plan, this recipe can be used as lunch and dinner. Any leftovers (the serving size is quite generous) can be used cold in a salad or added to an egg omelet the next day.

Nutrition Analysis (per serving size of 414 g):

Calories 430; Fat 10 g; Cholesterol 135 mg; Carbohydrates 12 g; Protein 56 g.

Adapted from It Must Be My Metabolism by Reza Yavari, MD (recipe by Jacques Pepin)

Chicken Adobo

Ingredients

3 lbs	Boneless chicken breast
½ cup	Red wine vinegar
½ cup	Soy sauce
2 cups	Chicken broth or water
1 leaf	Bay leaf
1 tbsp	Adobo herb mixture
2 cloves	Garlic, minced (or more to taste)
1 to 3 tbsp	Cornstarch or tapioca flour (optional)

Instructions

1. Mix all ingredients (except chicken and cornstarch) in large saucepan or Dutch oven and bring to boil.

2. When mixture is boiling, add chicken.

3. Reduce heat and simmer, covered, for 30 minutes.

4. Uncover and continue simmering for another half hour or until done.

Nutritional Analysis

per 6 ounce serving: 41 gm Protein, 210 Calories. Serves about 8.

per 4 ounce serving: 28 gm Protein, 140 Calories. Serves about 12

Celery Chickpea Stew with Chicken

Ingredients

2 to 2.5 lbs Chicken Thighs skinless, boneless; cut into halves
2 bunches   Celery, chopped in 1-inch pieces
2 medium   Onion, sliced coarsely
1 can   Chickpea (organic), drained and rinsed
1 bunch   Parsley (Italian or flat)
2 tbsp   Olive oil
2 tbsp   Tomato Paste
2 tbsp   Smoked Paprika
2 tbsp   Herbs de France
1 tbsp   Ancho or Guajillo Chili powder – (optional)
6 medium   Dried Limes – washed and gently crushed
2 tsp   Salt

Instructions

1. Cut 1 inch from either end of celery bunches, wash well.
2. With a sharp knife cut into 1-inch long pieces. If the bottom pieces are too thick cut them lengthwise.
3. Cut each onion into 2 halves then slice each half into ½ inch-wide slices.
4. Heat 1 tbsp of olive oil in a deep pan or skillet.
5. Add onions and celery to the pan.
6. Mix well and sauté at medium temperature for about 30 minutes or till onions are soft and celery pieces are slightly browned.
7. Mix often so the bottom pieces do not burn.
8. While vegetables are cooking, heat 1 tbsp of olive oil in a big heavy pot or a Dutch oven.
9. Place the chicken thighs one by one in the pot.
10. Generously cover both sides of chicken thighs pieces with Smoked Paprika.
11. Cook at medium temperature till chicken is browned on both sides.
12. Add additional seasoning such as salt and Herbs de France blend as well as chili powder, cook another 5 minutes to blend in spices.
13. Then add vegetables to the pot and mix well.

14. Add 2 cups of chicken broth, chickpeas and 2 tbsp of tomato paste (for color) and dried limes.

15. Mix and cook at low-medium for about 30 minutes, stirring every 10 minutes with a wooden spoon so the bottom does not burn.

16. Add chopped parsley 5-10 minutes before serving.

This is a very simple yet satisfying dish and can be reheated, consumed several times before eventually frozen for future meals (freeze in small containers.) If dried limes are difficult to find can add tamarind paste or even lemon juice to taste. You may wish to have a serving of white rice or cauli-rice with this stew. This is a very low-calorie dish and yet provides plenty of protein.

Nutrition Analysis: Estimated per serving (1/8): Calories 333; Protein 37 grams.

Cajun Chicken Avocado Pineapple Salad

Ingredients

3 lbs	Chicken Breast – boneless tenders

Cajun Spice Blend – use as needed

2 tbsp	Olive Oil
2 whole	Avocado, cut in cubes
2 tbsp	Salsa – mild or medium hot
4-6 tbsp	Cilantro, chopped
½	Ripe Pineapple, peeled, cubed (about 2 cups)
1 tbsp	Lemon Juice
1 tbsp	White Vinegar

Instructions

1. First broil the chicken tenders:
2. Add 1 tbsp of olive oil to chicken tenders in a big bowl and mix.
3. Add 1 tbsp (or more if desired) of Cajun blend to chicken tenders while mixing so strips are uniformly covered with spice mix.
4. Heat an oven-resistant platter or skillet with 1 tbsp of oil.
5. Place tenders in rows, about 4 inches below the broiler.
6. Cook at 400° for 10 minutes then turn over the strips. Cook for another 5 minutes or till slightly browned. Set aside.
7. (Cut one tender in half. Cooked chicken breast should not be shiny and should not be chewy. If not cooked enough, broil for an additional 5 minutes.
8. Cut avocado into cubes or slices.
9. Add pineapple cubes (pineapple has lots of sugar so if it is not recommended, it can be replaced with an apple or jicama strips)
10. Add chicken strips – roughly 4-6 strips per serving and refrigerate the rest.
11. Add white vinegar, lemon juice.
12. Toss and salt to taste.
13. Garnish with chopped cilantro.

Could be used later in tacos.

Nutrition Analysis:

Estimated per serving size: Calories 400; Protein 44 grams.

Broiled Chicken on Vegetable Salad

Ingredients

2 tbsp Finely chopped fresh tarragon leaves

1 1/2 tbsp Grated lemon rind

3/4 tsp Freshly ground black pepper

6 oz Skinless, boneless chicken breasts

Vegetable cooking spray

6 cups (loose) shredded iceberg lettuce

2 1/2 cups Peeled, seeded, and diced (1/2 inch) cucumbers

3 cups Washed and diced (1/2 inch) button mushrooms

2 cups Diced (3/4 inch) tomatoes

2 cups Peeled, diced potatoes, boiled in water to cover until tender

3 tbsp Extra virgin olive oil

1 tbsp Red wine vinegar

1 tbsp Dijon-style mustard

1/2 teaspoon salt

1/2 tbsp Freshly ground black pepper

2 tbsp Chopped chives or parsley leaves, for garnish

Instructions

This is a dish that could be divided, with the vegetables served separately from the meat, which is very flavorful served on its own this way. And, for a meatless lunch, the vegetable salad alone is a perfect choice. Any leftover chicken can be sliced and served cold the following day on greens with a little mustard. The cold chicken would also go well with a jalapeño dip.

1. Combine the tarragon, lemon, and 3/4 teaspoon pepper in a small bowl, and rub the mixture into both sides of the chicken breasts. Then spray the breasts lightly on both sides with the cooking spray.

2. Heat the broiler.

3. Arrange the chicken breasts side by side on a broiler rack, and place the pan so the chicken is about 4 inches from the heat.

4. Broil the chicken for approximately 4 minutes on each side. Set it aside to cool slightly while you assemble the salad.

5. Combine the lettuce, cucumbers, mushrooms, tomatoes, and potatoes in a large bowl.

6. Toss with the oil, vinegar, salt. and 1/2 teaspoon pepper.

7. Divide the salad among 6 dinner plates.

8. Cut each chicken breast in half on the diagonal and arrange 2 halves on top of the vegetable salad on each plate.

9. Garnish with the chopped chives or parsley, dividing it among the plates. Serve.

Nutrition Analysis (per serving size of 435 g): Calories 330; Fat 10 g; Cholesterol 100 mg; Carbohydrates 17; Protein 43 g. *Adapted from It Must Be My Metabolism by Reza Yavari, MD (recipe by Jacques Pepin)*

Black Bean Salsa with Chicken and Avocado Lettuce Tacos

Ingredients

Black Bean Salsa

2 large Poblano Peppers

2 Jalapeno Peppers

1 large or 2 medium Red Onion, chopped into small squares

2 cloves Fresh Garlic, minced

1 can Cooked Organic Black Beans, drained and rinsed

1 can Organic Diced Tomato

2 tsp Cumin Seeds (crushed) or Powder

2 tsp Salt, may adjust to taste later

Juice of 2 Limes

Fresh Cilantro chopped

2 tbs Olive oil

1 cup Vegetable Broth

Instructions

1. Cut peppers in halves lengthwise, remove seeds

2. Roast in oven at high temperature (450 +) for about 10 minutes or until skin is browned

3. Peel and chop (remove skin in cold water – optional)

4. In a non-stick pan heat olive oil then add chopped onion, peppers and garlic.

5. Cook at medium temperature until onions are slightly translucent – do not brown

6. Add dice tomatoes, mix.

7. Add black beans and mix.

8. Simmer in 1 cup of vegetable broth for about 15 minutes or until tomato pieces and beans are just soft.

9. Adjust salt.

10. Add lime juice and garnish with cilantro.

11. Divide into six servings.

12. Plate each serving on 3 lettuce leaves.

13. Add 2 strips of previously cooked boneless, skinless chicken breast to each leaf (approximately 1 oz per chicken breast strip).

14. Top with avocado slices and cilantro garnish.

15. Add salt and hot sauce to taste.
16. May serve warm or cold.

Nutrition Analysis:

Estimated per servings of 3 lettuce tacos: Calories 450; Protein 39 grams.

RECIPES: BEEF

Carne Molida with Jicama – Ground Beef Hash
Ingredients
2 lbs		Ground Beef (90% fat)
1 medium	Onion, diced
2 medium	Carrots, sliced
2 tbsp		Tomato Paste
2 cloves	Garlic
1 cup		Jicama, cubed
15		Pitted Olives, diced
4 tbsp		Sofrito
2 tbsp		Olive oil
1 tsp		Cumin
2 tsp		Ancho Pepper
½ cup		Cilantro, chopped
1 cup		Broth – prefer beef bone broth
Sofrito:
2 tbsp		Olive oil
4		Green Peppers, seeds and ribs removed, chopped
2		Red Bell peppers, seeds and ribs removed, chopped
2 large		Tomatoes, cut
2 medium	Onions, chopped

2 cloves	Garlic, chopped
1 batch	Cilantro, chopped
½ tsp	Salt

Instructions

1. Place all sofrito ingredients in a blender to puree.
2. Pour extra sofrito into small containers and keep frozen till ready to use.
3. Sauté diced onion and garlic in olive oil and sofrito – medium temperature for about 5 minutes or until onions become soft.
4. Add beef and carrot slices and mix well with onion garlic mix.
5. Add cumin, pepper, olives and brown for 5 minutes.
6. Add tomato paste, broth and jicama cubes.
7. Bring to a simmer, cover and cook till jicama is soft – may add more broth.
8. Salt to taste.
9. Garnish with chopped cilantro.

Nutrition Analysis:

Estimated per serving size of (1/6 or about 5 oz of meat): Calories 466; Protein 40 grams.

Beef Steak with Herb Crust

Ingredients

1 tsp Dried thyme

1 tsp Dried savory

1 large New York strip steak, about 1 1/2 pounds, trimmed of all fat (1 1/4 pounds trimmed weight)

1/2 tsp Freshly ground black pepper

1/2 Salt

1 TBSP Good olive oil

1/4 homemade chicken stock or low-salt canned chicken broth

Instructions

The best steak for me is the New York strip, which is also called a shell steak or loin steak. It is important to let the meat rest in a warm place after cooking, so it will be pink throughout. Cut into thin slices, a steak this size will serve 4 people with the addition of a salad and/or a couple of cooked vegetables. Any leftover steak is great sliced thin and served with a salad.

1. Heat the oven to 450 degrees.

2. Crush the dried herbs between your thumb and finger and mix them with the pepper in a small bowl. Pat the mixture on both sides of the meat.

3. When ready to cook, sprinkle the meat with the salt.

4. Heat the oil on top of the stove in a heavy ovenproof skillet or saucepan. When hot, add the meat, and cook over medium to high heat for 3 minutes on each side.

5. Transfer the steak to the preheated oven and cook for about 8 minutes for medium rare meat.

6. Remove the meat to a platter and let rest in a warm place for about 10 minutes before serving.

7. Add the stock to the drippings in the skillet and bring to a boil.

8. Cut the steak into thin slices and serve with the skillet juices spooned over them.

Nutrition Analysis (per serving size of 159 g):

Calories 320; Fat 16 g; Cholesterol 110 mg; Carbohydrates 1 g; Protein 41 g

Adapted from It Must Be My Metabolism by Reza Yavari, MD (recipe by Jacques Pepin)

Beef Picadillo Breakfast Burritos

Ingredients

1 lb	Ground Beef
1 large	Red Onion, chopped
1	Bell Pepper, chopped
2	Jalapenos, seeds and ribs removed, chopped
3 cloves	Garlic, minced
1 tbsp	Smoked Paprika
1 tbsp	Chili Powder (mild)
1 tbsp	Ground Cumin
1 tbsp	Oregano Dried
½ cup	Raisins, coarsely chopped
½ cup	Pimento Stuffed Green Olives, coarsely chopped
2 tbsp	Capers in Brine
2 tbsp	White wine vinegar
2 tbsp	Olive oil
2 tbsp	Salt
4	Egg whites
2	Whole eggs
6	10 inch Flour tortillas
6 oz	Mexican white cheese (Oaxaca part skim)

Cilantro; Hot sauce

Instructions

This is truly a breakfast for "champions on the go." Burritos may be prepared in advance and kept frozen. Microwave heated in a couple of minutes and a delicious breakfast. This Argentinian picadillo, like beef hash, may also be used in sandwiches, stews as well as empanadas.

In a large skillet heat olive oil, add onion, pepper, jalapenos and cook over medium heat. until onions pieces are translucent.

1. Add garlic, cook for 2-3 minutes while adding beef in chunks.

2. Mix chopped vegetables evenly with a wooden spoon.

3. Add spices and herbs one by one while mixing.

4. Add raisins, olives and capers and brown beef thoroughly for 20 minutes.

5. Add wine vinegar, mix and cook for another 3-5 minutes. Salt to taste.

6. Remove pan and set aside. May refrigerate for later use

7. Make scrambled eggs with 4 egg whites and 2 whole egg - salt to taste

8. Heat a burrito size flour tortilla on a dry pan for 30 seconds.

9. Add 1/6 of the picadillo to a 10-inch burrito flour tortilla, add 1/6 of egg scramble and 1 oz. shredded Mexican white cheese (Oaxaca part skim) and wrap tortilla into a burrito

10. Garnish with chopped cilantro and hot sauce to taste.

Nutrition Analysis: Estimated per burrito: Calories 565 (454 in Pita pocket); Protein 35 grams.

Beef Burgundy

Ingredients

1/2 lbs Beef stew meat from the shoulder blade or shank, cut into 1 ½ to 2-inch cubes

2 tbsp Soy sauce

1 cup Homemade chicken stock or low-salt canned chicken broth

1 1/2 cups Dry, fruity red wine

1 cup Peeled and chopped onion

1 tbsp Peeled, crushed, and finely chopped garlic

3/4 tsp Salt

1/4 tsp Freshly ground black pepper

2 Bay leaves

1/2 tsp Dried thyme leaves

About 18 medium button mushrooms

2 cups Carrots, peeled, halved, and diced (1 inch)

18 Small pearl onions, peeled

1 tbsp Cornstarch dissolved in 2 tablespoons water

1/2 cup Frozen petite peas, thawed

2 tbsp Chopped fresh parsley

Instructions

This classic beef burgundy is best made with either beef shank or shoulder blade. These cuts are lean and usually quite gelatinous, and they work well—much better than a piece of bottom or top round, which would be too dry. This type of stew always good to have on hand; the meat, can be cooked with the onion and wine and frozen, then heated at the last moment, with fresh vegetables added at the end. The stew is good served with most any starch, from pasta to potatoes.

1. Put the meat in a Dutch oven and add the soy sauce. Mix well.

2. Add the stock, wine, onion, garlic, salt, pepper, bay leaves, and thyme. Mix well. Bring to a strong boil over high heat, reduce the heat to low, cover, and boil very gently for 1 1/4 hours, or until the meat is tender.

3. Add the mushrooms, carrots, and whole onions to the Dutch oven, moving the meat in the pan with tongs to make room for the vegetables, and bring the mixture back to a boil.

4. Reduce the heat to low, cover, and boil very gently for 10 minutes.

5. Remove and discard the bay leaf and stir in the dissolved cornstarch mixture and the peas.

6. Bring the stew back to a boil, and serve, dividing the meat and vegetables among 6 plates.

7. Garnish each serving with a little of the parsley.

As part of your meal plan, this recipe can be used as a dinner or lunch.

Nutrition Analysis (per serving size of 478 g):

Calories 380; Fat 8 g; Cholesterol 75 mg; Carbohydrates 20; Protein 46 g.

Adapted from It Must Be My Metabolism by Reza Yavari, MD (recipe by Jacques Pepin)

RECIPES: FISH & SEAFOOD

Salmon Mango Salsa

Ingredients

Mango Salsa

1	Mango, chopped
1	Jalapeno, seeds and ribs removed, chopped
1 medium	Red onion, chopped
2 tbsp	Cilantro, chopped
2 tbsp	Lime Juice
½ tsp	Salt
½ tsp	Sugar
1 medium	Salmon filet (about 1.5 lbs; avoid pond-raised)
½ cup	Lemon Juice
2 tsp	Salt
1 tbsp	Olive oil

Instructions

1. Mix mango salsa ingredients well and set aside at room temperature or keep in refrigerator for later use. (Can make more by doubling every ingredient.)
2. Marinate salmon in lemon juice while heating oven to 400° - Do not marinate in lemon juice longer than 10 minutes.

3. Remove salmon and let lemon juice drain.
4. Heat 1 tbsp of olive oil in an oven-resistant platter or a deep skillet.
5. Place salmon in the container, add a pinch of salt and cover with generous spoonfuls of mango salsa.
6. Cover with aluminum foil and cook for 30 minutes.
7. Remove top and broil 4 inches below for another 5 to 10 minutes until slightly crisp on top.
8. Leftover salmon could be reheated and / or used in tacos or on top of a salad.

Nutrition Analysis:
Estimated per serving size: Calories 400; Protein 36 grams.

Ceviche of Scallops - Shrimp Tostada

Ingredients

1 lbs	Sea scallops or shelled small shrimp (Scallops washed and cut into 1-inch pieces)
1 cup	Red onion, diced (1/4-inch)
1 ½ cups	Tomato, diced (1/2-inch)
1	Jalapeño chili pepper, seeds and ribs removed, chopped
¼ cup	Cilantro, coarsely chopped
1	ime, julienned rind
¼ cup	Lime Juice
1 tbsp	White wine vinegar
2 tbsp	Mint, fresh, coarsely chopped
1 tsp	Salt
½ tsp	Pepper, freshly ground
2 tsp	Sugar
1	Cucumber, trimmed and peeled
8	Lettuce leaves size of a tortilla or fried corn tortilla patted dry (to remove extra oil)

Instructions

Ceviche is a South American—particularly Peruvian—type of marinated fish. The fish is "cooked" with citric acid from limes or lemons, Here, we use scallops or alternatively shrimp or a 50/50 mix of both. We extend the recipe by adding diced tomatoes, cilantro, mint, and a julienne of lime skin, which give the dish a zesty and piquant flavor. Diced cucumber, added at the end, adds some crunchiness and contrast. You can add julienne of jalapeño if you want heat. This dish is excellent as a first course, served on a plate or on pan fried corn tortillas. You could extend the recipe by adding additional fish, perhaps a dice of salmon or cod or add avocado slices. Always marinate the raw sea food in lime or lemon juice for a couple of hours. If you leave sea food in citric acid for too long, it becomes chewy and dehydrated.

1. Combine all the ingredients, except the cucumber, in a bowl.

2. Cover, and refrigerate for a couple of hours, stirring occasionally, so the mixture is well combined.

3. Cut the cucumber in half lengthwise and scrape out the seeds with a metal measuring spoon.

4. Cut the cucumber flesh into a 1/2-inch dice.

5. At serving time, mix the cucumber with the scallops, and divide the ceviche among 4 plates.

Nutrition Facts (per serving of 4 ounces of scallops or shrimp or 2 tostadas):

Total protein about 28 g; 180 calories if served on two lettuce leaves.

If served on fried corn tortillas add 200 calories (100 calories per fried corn tortilla.)

Adapted from It Must Be My Metabolism by Reza Yavari, MD (recipe by Jacques Pepin.)

Marinated Squid Vietnamese-Style

Ingredients

1 lbs Squid (body and tentacles), thoroughly cleaned

1 tbsp Peeled, crushed, and finely chopped garlic

1 tsp Seeded and chopped Thai hot chili peppers

1 1/2 cups Very thinly sliced onion

2 tbsp Lime juice

1/3 cup Shredded fresh mint

1/3 cup Coarsely chopped fresh cilantro leaves

3 tbsp *nuoc nam* (Vietnamese fish sauce)

1/2 tsp Sugar

4 Large iceberg lettuce leaves

Instructions

This dish, a kind of ceviche, is inspired by a Vietnamese style of cooking. Notice that there is no oil in this dish; the combination of hot chili peppers (use whatever variety you prefer, and less or more, depending on your tolerance for spicy food), mint, and cilantro creates a very fresh taste that goes well with the squid. This recipe can be served as the main course for a light lunch or, in smaller portions, as the first course for a dinner; you can shred more salad greens than I use here and serve the squid on the greens. Leftover squid is also good spooned over sliced avocado or diced fresh tomatoes.

1. Bring 6 cups of water to a boil in a large saucepan.

2. Cut the body pieces and tentacles of the squid crosswise into 1-inch slices.

3. Add the squid to the boiling water, and cook for about 2 minutes, stirring occasionally, until the water returns to the boil. Drain.

4. Combine the remaining ingredients, except the lettuce, in a large serving bowl. Add the hot, drained squid, and toss until well mixed.

5. Let marinate for at least 15 minutes, stirring occasionally, so the squid can develop flavor.

6. Serve on the lettuce leaves.

As part of your meal plan, this recipe can be used as part of a meal, a salad or as a snack.

Nutrition Analysis (per serving size of 199 g):
Calories 140; Fat 1.5g; Cholesterol 265 mg; Carbohydrates 10 g; Protein 19 g.

Adapted from It Must Be My Metabolism by Reza Yavari, MD (recipe by Jacques Pepin)

Jerk Scallops with Kale and White Beans

Ingredients

½ lb	Scallops, large (or about 10-12)
1 batch	Kale, washed, and leafy parts ripped off the veins and stems. Chopped into short strips.
1 can	Organic Cannellini Beans, drained and rinsed.
2 tbsp	Olive oil
½ tbsp	Butter (1 pat) (optional)
2 tbsp	Jerk Spice* Mix
2 tsp	Salt 2
2 oz	Dry white wine (optional)

Instructions

Almost all our recipes can be used as leftovers, reheated and/or added cold to salads. But NOT scallops. Scallops "do not keep" meaning you have to eat all of it in one meal. Scallops are also unique in that they are almost entirely made of protein. So, a smaller amount goes a long way in providing a high protein low calorie meal. Finally, it is also amazing how fast scallops cook. In fact, it is easy to overcook scallops into chewy and tasteless bites. Cook no longer that five minutes. We prefer larger scallops for main dishes. Smaller scallops (also called Bay Scallops) are better for mixed seafood dishes.

Ten to twelve large scallops weigh about half a pound. Each large of scallop has about 5 grams of protein for only 25 calories – that is about as lean as a natural protein can get. When buying large scallops, you may ask for a dozen large ones (two servings). If you buy them frozen in a bag, then count about 5 to 6 per person.

1. Rinse scallops, drain and then mix with 1 tbs of olive oil in a medium size bowl.

2. Add Jerk spice mix until all scallops are evenly seasoned. Set aside.

3. In a heavy skillet heat 1 tbs of olive oil.

4. Add kale and heat at medium temperature until soft - about 5 minutes.

5. Add 1 tsp of salt.

6. Add beans and mix.

7. Heat for another 10 minutes – may add some water or broth for moisture.

8. Remove vegetables from pan.

9. Add scallops to the same pan and cook for about 5 minutes at medium high turning scallops once.

10. In the last minute may add 2 ounces of dry white wine for glazing.

11. Add butter (optional) and serve immediately.

12. Salt to taste.

If you want to eat more protein increase scallop portions and cut back on beans (1 large scallop has about 5 grams of protein.)

*Jerk Spice Mix can be purchased online, at specialty spice stores or at most supermarkets.

Nutrition Analysis: Estimated per serving of about 5-6 scallops with half of kale / beans mixture cooked as described above: Calories 370; Protein 30 grams; Carbs 10 grams.

Halibut with Fennel and Orange Slices

Ingredients

2 lbs or 2 fillets	Halibut
2 bulbs	Fennel, remove bottom ½ inch then slice thin or shave; chop leaves and save for garnish
1	Orange – peeled, sliced with a sharp blade from stem to blossom end into about 10 tranches,
1 tbsp	Jerk Herb Mix
1 tsp	Salt
1 cup	Lemon Juice
1 tbsp	Olive oil

Instructions

1. Marinate halibut fillets in lemon juice for no longer than 10 minutes.
2. Remove and drain, add herb mixture and salt (could add any other seasoning of your choice.)
3. Heat oven to 400°.
4. Heat a medium size oven resistant platter with 1 tbsp olive oil spread evenly then place orange slices at the bottom.
5. Place fennel slices on top. Then lay fillets on top of fennel slices.
6. Bake for about 25-30 minutes.
7. Garnish with chopped fennel leaves.
8. Divide into 4 and serve all layers with a spatula.

Could reheat remaining leftover or mince fillets for fish tacos.

Nutrition Analysis:

Estimated per serving size (about 6 oz): Calories 190; Protein 36 grams.

RECIPES: TURKEY

Argentinian Style Turkey Picadillo

Ingredients

1 lb	Ground turkey
1 large	Red onion, chopped
1	Bell Pepper, chopped
2	Jalapenos, seeds and ribs removed, chopped
3 cloves	Garlic, minced
1 tbsp	Smoked paprika
1 tbsp	Chili powder (mild)
1 tbsp	Ground cumin
1 tbsp	Dried oregano
½ cup	Raisins, coarsely chopped
½ cup	Pimento Stuffed Green Olives, coarsely chopped
2 tbsp	Capers in Brine
2 tbsp	White wine vinegar
2 tbsp	Olive oil
2 tbsp	Salt

Instructions

1. In a large skillet heat olive oil, add onion, pepper, jalapenos

and cook over medium heat. until onions pieces are translucent.
2. Add garlic, cook for 2-3 minutes while adding turkey in chunks.
3. Mix chopped vegetables evenly with a wooden spoon.
4. Add spices and herbs one by one while mixing.
5. Add raisins, olives and capers and brown turkey thoroughly for 20 minutes.
6. Add wine vinegar, mix and cook for another 3-5 minutes. (May add broth to keep moist – optional)
7. Salt to taste.
8. Remove pan and set aside. May refrigerate for later use.

This is an Argentinian style turkey picadillo that is often used for empanadas. But picadillo like beef hash may be used in many different ways such as burritos, sandwiches, stews as well as empanadas. This recipe uses turkey but feel free to use ground beef. Serves 4.

Nutrition Analysis:

Estimated per serving size (serves 4): Calories 300; Protein 20 grams.

Turkey Chili

Ingredients

1 lbs	Ground Turkey
1 can	Black beans – drained and rinsed
1 can	Red beans – drained and rinsed
1 large can	Diced tomatoes – (Glen Muir)
1 medium to large Onion, chopped	
1	Bell pepper - seeds and ribs removed, chopped
1	Jalapeno – seeds and ribs removed, chopped
3 cloves	Garlic, minced
1 tsp	Salt
1 tsp	Black pepper
½ tsp	Oregano – dried
½ tsp	Chili powder (optional)
½ cup	Broth
2 tbsp	Olive oil

Instructions

1. In a deep skillet or a heavy pot sauté onion and Bell pepper at medium high temperature till onion is soft (about 10 minutes) stirring a few times.

2. Add chopped jalapeño, garlic and turkey in 1-inch chunks and mix well.

3. Heat for 5 minutes and stir again.

4. Add tomatoes, oregano and stir well. Cook at medium for 30 to 45 minutes.

5. May add ½ cup vegetable or chicken broth for additional liquid - if need be.

6. Add salt and pepper to taste. To increase pepper heat may add chili powder to taste.

Nutrition Analysis:

Estimated per serving size (serves 4): Calories 400; Protein 34 grams.

RECIPES: PORK

Smoked Pork with Honey Glaze

Ingredients

1   Smoked picnic pork shoulder with bone in (about 6 pounds)

2 tbsp Honey

2 tsp Dry mustard

2 tbsp Chinese hot chili and garlic paste

1 cup Chicken stock

Instructions

This is an ideal dish to prepare over a weekend when you are entertaining; it's easy to do and tasty, and the guests can help themselves. The cooking of the pork shoulder roast in water removes a lot of its salt and smokiness and preserves the moisture in the meat. The best part of the dish for me, however, is the leftovers. The meat makes a great sandwich filling with mustard and it's delicious served alongside eggs in the morning. Also, there is nothing better than little pieces of the meat mated with vegetables or pasta and reheated in a gratin dish. Even the leftover bone can be re-boiled to create a stock that you can freeze and use later to make a soup with split peas or beans.

1. Put the pork shoulder in a stockpot and add enough cold water to extend about 1/2 inch above the meat.

2. Bring the water to 180 degrees (just below the boil) and cook for 1 1/2 hours at this temperature.
3. Meanwhile, make the glaze: Mix the honey, mustard, and hot chili paste together in a small bowl.
4. Heat the oven to 400 degrees.
5. Let the pork cool in the cooking liquid, then cut off and discard the exterior fat and the rind from around the bones.
6. Score the top of the ham, cutting intersecting lines about 1/2-inch-deep into it every 3/4-inch. Spread the glaze over the surface.
7. Put the pork in a roasting pan and bake in the preheated oven for 1 hour. The surface should be nicely browned.
8. Transfer the pork to a serving platter and set aside in a warm place.
9. Add the chicken stock to the pan juices and stir with a wooden spoon to dissolve any solidified juices.
10. Strain the juices over the pork shoulder, cut into slices, and serve.

As part of your meal plan, this recipe can be used as a meal, in a salad or with eggs for breakfast.

Nutrition Analysis (per serving size of 139 g):
Calories 270; Fat 15 g; Cholesterol 105 mg; Carbohydrates 4 g; Protein 29 g.

Adapted from It Must Be My Metabolism by Reza Yavari, MD (recipe by Jacques Pepin)

Puerto Rican Pork Roast

Ingredients

4-5 lbs	Pork shoulder - trim excess fat off
3 tbsp	Adobo spice blend
3 tbsp	White or cider vinegar
1 tbsp	Salt
1 tbsp	Black pepper
1 tbsp	Chili powder, mild such as Ancho or Guajillo
4 tbsp (1/4 cup)	Olive oil
8-10 cloves	Garlic

Instructions

This is a dish that takes time to cook but requires little work. Once cooked it may be consumed many times over, reheated, shredded for sandwiches and tacos, etc. A bone-in pork shoulder weighing 4 lbs could take 3 to 4 hours to roast while a party size 8-pound piece could easily take 6 hours. In addition, most recipes call for the pork to be marinated at least overnight or longer. So, we suggest this recipe for weekend batch cooking and for parties.

1. Press minced garlic and mix with olive oil, vinegar, Adobo mix, chili powder, salt and pepper. Set paste aside.
2. Remove excess fat from pork shoulder.
3. Make many deep (1 inch) cuts in the meat to the bone (every inch or so) using a small knife.
4. Stuff slits with paste and rub remainder of it on pork skin.
5. Place the shoulder in a large plastic bag and refrigerate overnight.
6. Next day bring to room temperature for 1-2 hours prior to roasting.
7. Heat oven to 300°, place shoulder in a roasting pan with a rack.
8. Cook for 4 hours turning sides every hour.
9. Turn roast skin-side up and raise temperature to 400° in the last 30 minutes to get crispy skin.
10. Take out and leave at room temperature for 15 to 30 minutes before serving.

Nutrition Analysis:

Estimated per serving: Calories 350; Protein 32 grams.

Pork Adobo Filipino Style

Ingredients

1 cup	Wine vinegar
½ cup	Soy sauce (low sodium)
2 cups	Water
2	Bay leaf
2 cloves	Garlic, minced
1	Jalapeno, seeds and ribs removed, minced
3 lbs	Pork chunks
2 tbs	Cornstarch or Tapioca (optional used as thickener)

Instructions

1. Mix all ingredients (except meat and cornstarch) in large saucepan or Dutch oven and bring to boil.

2. When mixture is boiling, add meat.

3. Reduce heat and simmer, covered, for 30 minutes.

4. Uncover and continue simmering for another half hour or until done.

If you want the liquid to be thicker, add cornstarch and stir gently. Meat tends to "fall apart" so do not over-agitate during cooking process or when adding cornstarch. Remove bay leaf before serving.

Nutritional Analysis:

Estimated per 6 ounce serving: Calories 290; Protein 39 grams.

Citrus Marinated Adobo Pork Chops with Apples

Ingredients

6	Pork chops center-cut (about 2 lbs trimmed of fat)
2 tbsp	Adobo spice mix
½ cup	Tomatillo hot sauce – mild
½ cup	Orange juice
2 tbsp	Dijon mustard
2 tbsp	Honey
2	Apples, peeled, cored and sliced - Golden Delicious or Honey-crisp
1 tbsp	Olive oil

Instructions

1. In a medium size bowl mix tomatillo sauce, mustard, honey and orange juice.

2. Stir well and set aside.

3. Rub both sides of chops with generous amounts of Adobo spice.

4. Heat olive oil in a large non-stick pan add pork chops and fry one side at medium hot temperature for 5 minutes or till browned.

5. Turn over chops, lower heat to medium and brown the other side for 5 minutes.

6. Add citrus marinade and cook for an additional 5 minutes.

7. Remove chops to a platter and keep warm.

8. Add apple slices to the pan and cook in citrus sauce till apple slices turn soft.

9. Stir apple slices in sauce to make a puree.

10. Pour puree over chops and serve.

A side dish of sautéed mushrooms with leafy greens would complete this dish. (This recipe appears to have lots of sugar, but it only has about 30 grams of sugar total - from honey, orange juice and apple - that is 10 grams or less per serving.)

Nutrition Analysis:

Estimated per serving (2 chops) – sauce included: Calories 380; Protein 46 grams.

Serving Size is 2 chops. If a serving of 2 chops is too much meat add a side of white beans to the vegetable side dish and serve with one chop.

One chop with added white beans would yield about 30 grams of protein.

Size: Calories 446; Protein 22 grams

RECIPES: VEGETARIAN

Glazed Tofu
    Ingredients
    Medium Firm Tofu – 1 block of approximately of 15 ounces – drained
    Olive oil – 2 tbsp
    Paprika Smoked – 2 tbsp
    Coriander Seed Powder – 2 tbsp

Cut block of tofu into 5 slices each about 1.5 cm thick. Place on 2 layers of paper towel and cover with 2 layers to drain for about 10 minutes.

Heat oil in a medium non stick pan at medium temperature for 2 minutes.

Remove paper towels and cut each slice into 4 rectangles. Cover the top surface of tofu rectangles with paprika. Place them paprika face down in heated oil and fry for 2-3 minutes. Add coriander powder and flip rectangles over (coriander surface down now) and fry for an additional 2 minutes. May add white wine and cook for 1-2 minutes (optional.)

Remove and set aside. Glazed tofu is then added to many other recipes such as stews or salads. When serving, it is easier to keep track of nutrition content per rectangle.

Nutrition Analysis:

1 block of tofu is usually about 1 pound of 14 ounces drained. 1 lbs of tofu is about 350 calories and contains 40 grams of protein.

Each block is cut into 20 rectangles. Each rectangle has about 17.5 calories for 2 grams of protein.

Therefore, a serving size of 8 rectangles provides about 15 grams of protein for 140 calories.

Glazed Tofu with Celery and Chickpea Stew

Serves 4

Ingredients

Glazed Tofu Medium Firm 1 block (see below)

Celery – 2 bunches

Chickpeas – 1 can (prefer organic)

Onions – 2 medium white, chopped

Tomato or Marinara Sauce– 2 cups

Cilantro – 1 bunch chopped

Olive oil – 2 tbsp

Vegetable Broth – 1 box or 4 cups

Coriander Seed Powder – 1 tbsp

Black Cumin – 1 tsp

Chili Powder – 1 tsp

Salt – 2 tsp

Cut celery at both ends by 1 inch and wash under running water. Then chop to 1-inch long pieces. Chop onions. In a large skillet or pot heat oil and add chopped onion and celery pieces and sauté at medium temperature till onions are soft and celery is slightly browned for about 10 minutes mixing every 3-4 minutes.

Add tomato marinara, chickpeas, spices and mix. Add broth, stir and cook at low-medium for 10 minutes. Add tofu on top and soak pieces in the stew. Add chopped cilantro. Cook an additional 10-15 minutes.

Nutrition Analysis:

Estimated per serving size: Calories 290; Protein 16 grams.

Tofu with Leeks, Chickpeas and Sun-dried Tomatoes- Serves 4
Ingredients
Tofu Medium Firm - 1 block or approximately 1 lbs
Hummus – 3 tbsp
Garlic – 3 cloves – chopped and crushed
Leeks – 2 medium slices thin
Chickpeas – 1 can (prefer organic) drained and rinced
Sun-dried Tomatoes – ¾ cup
Onion – 1 medium chopped
Swiss Cheese – 1 oz, grated
Jalapenos – 2 seeded and chopped
Olive oil –2 tbsp
Cumin – 1 tsp crushed or powdered
Paprika – 2 tsp
Coriander Seed Powder – 2 tsp
Salt – 2 tsp
Black Pepper – 1 tsp
(Mix spice blend and save.)
Turmeric – for color – 1 tsp (optional)
Panko Crumbs – 2 tbsp (optional)

Slice tofu in 1 cm slices and drain excess water with paper towels (15 minutes while preparing vegetables.) Then cut into cubes. Heat 1 tbsp of olive oil in a non-stick pan or skillet. Add chopped onion and jalapenos as well as chickpeas, leeks and sun dried tomatoes, mix. Add spice blend. Cook at medium temperature for 10 minutes – may add water or vegetable broth to keep moist. During this time pre-heat oven to 400 and blend tofu in a food processor with humus, salt and pepper. If tofu is too thick add water or broth. Spread 1 tbsp of olive oil in a platter. May add some turmeric for color and Panko crumbs for a thin crust (or use a pre-made frozen pie crust). Mix blended tofu with sautéed vegetable and cheese, add mixture to the platter. Spread to an even thickness and bake for 35-40 minutes.

Nutrition Analysis: Estimated Per Serving Size: Calories 446; Protein 22 grams.

Tofu with Butternut Squash and Chickpeas in Walnut Raison Apricot Pomegranate Sauce

Tofu Medium Firm – 1 block or approximately 1 lbs

Butternut Squash – Chopped, 1 container or 6 cups

Onions – 2 medium, chopped

Walnuts – 1.5 cup or 3 oz, crushed to crumbs in a plastic bag

Chickpeas – 1 can (prefer organic) drained and rinced

Raisons – ½ cup

Apricot Dry – 8-10 (optional)

Olive Oil – 1 tbsp

Honey – 1 tbsp

Pomegranate Molasse – 4 tbsp (heat bottle is a big bowl of hot water before pouring molasse into a container)

Cumin – 1 tsp crushed or powdered

Coriander Seed Powder – 2 tsp

Salt- 1 tsp

Vegetable Broth – 1 box or 3-4 cups

This delicious dish is more like a "party" dish. It is best consumed as a side dish with other sources of protein. Alternatively, the tofu portion can be increased to add extra protein with little additional calories.

Prepare glazed tofu as described previously.

In a large deep skillet, heat 1 tbsp of olive oil to medium temperature. Add chopped onion, butternut squash, walnut crumbs, chickpeas, raisons and apricots and sauté for 15 minutes at medium temperature, mixing evenly and stirring every 5 minutes. Add 4 tbsp of pomegranate molasse to 1 cup of broth and stir till mixed well. Add to it 1 tbsp of honey and stir well. Pour the mixture into the skillet and cook an additional 10 minutes at low temperature. If need be, add more broth to keep sauce thick but not dry.

Add tofu pieces to sauce, pour 1 cup of broth and add spice mixture. Cook for 5-10 minutes soaking tofu into sauce with a spatula.

Nutrition Analysis:

Estimated Per Serving: Calories 510; Protein 17 grams.

Three Bean Salad - Serves 6 – more as a side dish
Ingredients
Garbanzo Beans – 2 cans (prefer organic beans)
Cannellini Beans – 2 cans
Kidney Beans – 2 cans
Celery Stalk – 2, washed and chopped small
Jalapeno – 1 seeds and ribs removed, chopped small
Red Onion – 1 medium, chopped small
Flat Parsley – 1 cup chopped
Rosemary - 1 tsp chopped (or dry ground if fresh is not available)
Salt- 2 tsp

Empty all cans in a big colander or strainer, drain and rinse. Shake so all water is drained then transfer to a big bowl. Add chopped celery, jalapeno and onion. Mix with big spoons. Set aside.

Make salad dressing:
Lemon Juice – ½ cup
Wine Vinegar – 2 tbsp
Dijon Mustard – 2 tbsp
Garlic – 1 clove chopped and crushed
Salt- 1 tsp
Pepper – 1 tsp
Olive Oil – 3 tbsp

Scoop 2 tbsp of mustard into a measuring cup or a deep bowl. Add all ingredients except for oil and stir well till mustard is all dissolved. Add olive oil (if using in a measuring cup to a full cup if not add 3 tbsp) and stir well.

Pour the dressing (all of it or as desired depending how dry you wish the salad be) and mix well. Add parsley and rosemary and mix. Salt to taste. Cover, set aside at room temperature or refrigerate for an hour or longer.

If used as a side dish it is more than six servings.

Nutrition Analysis:
Estimated per serving: Calories 262; Protein 13 grams.

Mushroom and Apple Salad

With Cucumber-Yogurt Dressing

Yield: 6 servings

This is a great combination of ingredients, very refreshing as a light lunch or as a garnish to a grilled piece of meat or a roast turkey. The cucumber-yogurt dressing works well on most green salads and tomato salads but is also good spooned over grilled chicken or fish or cold chicken.

Cucumber-yogurt dressing

cup chunks of peeled and seeded cucumber
1/4 cup coarsely chopped scallions
tablespoon chopped fresh tarragon
cloves garlic, peeled
tablespoons fresh lime juice
tablespoons virgin olive oil
1/2 teaspoon salt
1 1/2 cups plain nonfat yogurt
2 1/2 cups sliced (1/2-inch) button mushrooms
2 apples, halved, cored, and cut into 1/2-inch dice
1/2 teaspoon salt
6 large Romaine lettuce leaves

For the cucumber-yogurt dressing: Put all the ingredients for the dressing, except the yogurt, in a blender, and blend until smooth. Transfer the mixture to a bowl and stir in the yogurt. (You will have about 2 cups.) Set aside 1 cup of the dressing for the salad, and store the remainder, tightly covered, in the refrigerator for up to 10 days to use on salads or grilled meat or fish.

Mix together the mushrooms, apples, salt, and reserved cup of dressing in a bowl. Arrange a lettuce leaf on each of 6 plates and spoon a heaping cup of the salad into each leaf. Serve.

Nutrition Analysis:

Estimated per serving size of about 200 grams: Calories 110; Protein 4 grams.

As part of your meal plan, this recipe can be used as a side dish, in a salad or as a snack.

Adapted from Jacques Pepin's recipe in *It Must Be My Metabolism* by R. Yavari, MD

Eggplant Split Pea and Tofu Stew - Serves 4

Ingredients

Tofu Medium Firm – 1 block or 1 lbs (see recipe for Glazed Tofu)

Eggplants – 3 medium sized or a total of 3 lbs, sliced into 1-inch thick circles

Onions – 4 medium whites, chopped

Split Peas – 1 cup

Tomato or Marinara Sauce – 2 cups

Olive Oil – 3 tbsp

Spice Mix Blend of your choice such All Spice – 2 tbsp

Turmeric – 2 tbsp

Chili Powder of your choice – prefer Gujaillo Powder – 2 tsp

Salt – 2 tsp

Vegetable Broth – 1 box or 4 cups

Boil water in a medium size pot. Wash and drain split peas and cook in boiling water for 15 minutes while heating oven to 400. In a large oven-resistant platter, spread 2 tbsp of olive oil. Divide each eggplant slice into 4-6 cubes, place in the platter and toss till all pieces are covered with oil. Then using a teaspoon to add turmeric to all pieces. Place in the heated oven for 15 minutes.

Remove split peas from stove and drain. Set aside.

Take eggplants out of oven and using a spatula, flip pieces over to cook the other sides. Roast for another 15 minutes till brown. Remove and set aside.

While roasting eggplants, heat 1 tbsp of oil in a skillet or a pot and sauté onions till soft. Drain split peas and add to onions. Add tomato sauce, spices and salt. Mix and cook for 5 minutes at medium temperature. Add eggplants and then add broth, gently stir. Let simmer for 15 minutes. Add glazed tofu (see recipe) to the stew and simmer for another 15 minutes. Salt to taste. Serve each plate with desired amount of eggplants and split peas as well as broth. In order to provide enough protein each serving should ideally have 4 to 6 cubes of tofu.

Nutrition Analysis:

Estimated per serving: Calories 517; Protein 28

Egg White Scramble with Veggie Patties
  Serves 1
  Ingredients

Egg Whites - 3
  Morningstar Farms Patties or another brand - 2
  Feta cheese – 1 oz, crumbled
  Salsa of your choice (mild) – 1 tbsp
  Sliced Tomato – 2
  Oregano – 1 tsp
  Salt – 1 tsp
  Black Pepper – 1 tsp

Lightly spray a non-stick pan with Pam or olive oil. Scramble egg whites with your choice of salsa. Salt and pepper to taste and set aside. Cook patties in pan for 2 minutes at medium high temperature (can place frozen patties directly on pan or first microwave for 30 seconds.) Flip patties over, put crumbled cheese on top and cook for another 2-3 minutes. Place tomato slices on top, sprinkle with oregano and serve with eggs.
  Nutrition Analysis:
  Estimated: Calories 350; Protein 40 grams.

Edamame Sesame Soba Noodle Bowl - Serves 4

This tasty dish is relatively low-carb and since soba noodle is made from buckwheat it is also gluten free.

Ingredients
Soba Noodles – 8 ounces
Edamame or Shelled Soybeans (frozen) – 1 package or 12 oz
Red Bell Pepper – 1, ribs and seeds removed and julienned
Red Cabbage – ½ sliced thin
Scallion – 1 bunch sliced thin
Sesame Seeds – 2 tsp
Sesame Oil (prefer toasted) – 1 tbsp
Soy or Soba Sauce – ½ cup
Salt – 1 tsp

Peanut Sauce Ingredients:
Peanut butter – 5 tbsp
Soy or Soba Sauce (also called soba soup base) – 5 tbsp
Sesame Oil (prefer toasted) – 2 tbsp
Honey – 1 tbsp
Siracha or other Chili Sauce – 1 tbsp
Lime or Lemon Juice – 1 tbsp
Add water if the sauce is too thick

Slowly add Soba noodles to a big pot of boiling water, turn down temperature and boil for 3-5 minutes (read package instructions for the exact time.) Then quickly drain hot water and dump noodles in a big bowl or pot of cold water. While soaking in cold water using your fingers separate noodles free of clumps. Drain water then add 1 tbsp of sesame oil and ½ cup of soy or soba sauce (or tamari if gluten-free), mix well and set aside.

Empty frozen edamame into a pot of boiling water. Add 1 tsp of salt and wait till water reboils then count 3-4 minutes. Taste the beans to make sure they are cooked (but do not let them get too soft.) Drain and set aside.

If the noodles and edamame are to be served hot, soak them in hot water for 5 minutes before mixing.

Mix in julienned bell pepper and cabbage strips with peanut sauce. Add to noodles and mix in edamame. Garnish with scallion and sesame seeds.

Nutrition Analysis: Estimated per serving size: Calories 540; Protein 21 grams

Black Bean Tostada – California Style

Serves 2

Ingredients

Corn Tortilla – 4

Black Beans Canned – organic – 1 can

Salsa – medium – 4 tbsp

Avocado – 1 ripe and sliced

Tomato – 1 large or 2 mediums – seeds removed, chopped

Red Onions – sliced thin marinated in lemon juice for 1 hour or longer

White Cheese – 2 oz, grated

Jalapenos 4-6 – seeded and sliced thin

Lettuce – 2 leaves shredded

First prepare black beans: Drain and boil for 30 minutes. Take about 1/3 and blend with 4 tbsp of salsa (about 4-6 pulses.) Add bean-salsa mix to beans, stir and salt. Set aside.

Brown 4 tortillas in vegetable oil – not hard but crispy; place on paper taper to remove excess oil.

Place tortillas on a cutting board or a tray. Add two large table spoons of black beans to each tortilla; spread evenly to cover the whole surface. Next add cheese, lettuce, chopped tomatoes, pickled onions and jalapeno slices.

Nutrition Analysis:

Estimated for a serving size of 2 tostadas: Calories 350; Protein 15 grams

Black Bean (Caraotas Negras) with Soy Sausage
  Serves 4
  Ingredients
  Black Beans – 2 cups canned organic
  Soy Links – 4 cut in 1 cm slices (Morning Star or similar organic brand)
  Bell Pepper – 1 chopped
  Poblano Peppers – 1, ribs and seeds removed, chopped
  Jalapeño Peppers – 1 medium or 2 small, ribs and seeds removed, chopped
  Onions – 2 medium chopped
  Garlic – 2 cloves chopped and crushed
  Vegetable Broth – 1 cup
  White Vinegar – 1 tbsp
  Olive Oil – 2 tbsp
  Cumin Powder – 2 tsp
  Cinnamon Powder – 1 tsp
  Coriander Powder – 2 tsp

Heat olive oil in a pan; mix chopped onion, peppers and sausage links and cook at medium temperature till onion are soft and sausage is slightly browned. Add black beans and spices. Pour in broth, add white vinegar and cook at low temperature for 15 to 20 minutes. Salt to taste.

When possible use dried black beans. You will have to bring to a boil and soak overnight. You may then have to boil at low temperature for 2 hours before adding to this recipe.

  Nutrition Analysis:
  Estimated per serving size: Calories 280; Protein 25 grams.

Artichoke Spinach & Mushroom Quiche
Serves 4
Ingredients
Spinach – 2 cups fresh (about 2 ounces)
Artichokes Frozen & Chopped – 3 cups (or a frozen package)
Mushrooms – 1 cup sliced
Onion – medium ½ chopped
Cheddar Cheese – 1 oz grated
Swiss Cheese – 1 oz grated
Eggs Whole – 2 whisked for 1 minute and set aside
Pie Crust Pre-Made Frozen – 1 nine inches
Olive Oil – 2 tbsp
Salt – 1 tsp
Pepper – 1 tsp
Cumin – 1 tsp crushed (optional)
Coriander Seed Powder – 1 tsp (optional)
Chili Powder – of your choice – 1 tsp (optional)

Pre-heat oven to 400. Heat 2 tbsp of olive oil in a large non-stick pan or skillet at medium temperature for 1 to 2 minutes. Sauté mushroom slices and chopped onion for 5-8 minutes or till onion pieces are translucent. Add spinach and artichoke, mix and cook till the pieces are slightly wilted and soft. Remove and pour into a bowl. Mix grated cheese with whisked eggs, add salt, pepper and spice blend, then pour into the bowl containing mushrooms. Mix well. Place the pie crust on an oven resistant platter. Add the quiche mix to the pie crust and spread evenly. Bake in heated oven for 50 to 60 minutes till browned on top (but not dry.) May add additional salt to taste

Nutrition Analysis:
Estimated Per Serving: Calories 349; Protein 20 grams.

RECIPES: SALADS & DIPS

Beluga Lentil Edamame and Roasted Tomato Salad
   Serves 8

Beluga or petite black lentils are less starchy than regular green lentils and hold up better in a salad.

   Ingredients
   Beluga Lentils – 2 cups
   Tomatoes – 8 medium Plum or Roma
   Edamame or Shelled Soy Beans – 1 frozen package or 12 oz
   Red Onion – 1 large, sliced think
   Feta or Goat or Gorgonzola Cheese (optional)
   Herb de Provence (or similar blend)
   Salt – 1 tsp
   Black Pepper – 1 tsp
   Olive Oil Spray
   Mustard Vinaigrette Salad Dressing – 2 to 4 tbsp

Heat oven to 400. Place 8 tomatoes (may cut in halves and place them skin up) in an oven resistant platter and spray with olive oil.

Roast for about 40 minutes. Remove and set aside.

While tomatoes are roasting bring a pot of water to boil and gently pour the lentils in the water. Bring to boil again then lower temperature and cook for 30 minutes. Lentils should be soft but not mushy (even a little chewy is better.) Drain and set aside. Heat water to boil then add frozen edamame. Bring to boil and cook for a about 5 minutes. Beans should also be soft but not mushy.

Mix onion slices, lentils and beans then add to roasted tomatoes. Sprinkle with crumbled cheese (optional.) May refrigerate for several days.

When ready to serve add salad dressing as desired (additional mustard may be used for extra punch.) Salt and pepper to taste.

Nutrition Analysis:

Estimated per serving: Calories 200; Protein 18 grams

(Does not include the dressing and optional cheese)

Spinach Cucumber Apple and Yogurt Salad
Ingredients
Spinach – 1 bunch or as needed (prefer organic), wash and water
English Cucumber – 1 peeled and sliced thin
Apple – ½ peeled and sliced (prefer a tart apple)

Yogurt – 1 cup, plain, whole or low fat, organic
Extra Virgin Olive Oil - ½ tbsp
Mint – Dry, ½ tbsp
Oregano – Dry, ½ tbsp
Salt – 1 tsp

Mix yogurt sauce well and salt to taste. Add cucumber and apple slices to spinach and toss. Add as much sauce as desired and toss again. Serve generously or as much as you wish.

Nutrition Analysis:
Not a major source of calories or protein.

Roasted Chickpeas and Turkish Salad Spice
Serves 4

Ingredients

Chickpeas (aka Garbanzo Beans) – 2 cans (prefer organic), drain and rinse
Olive Oil – 1 tbsp

Turkish Salad Spice:
   Sumac – 2 tbsp
   Chili Powder – 1 tsp
   Oregano Dry – 2 tsp
   Cumin Powder or Crushed – 1 tsp
   Salt – 1 tsp
   Garlic Powder – 1 tsp

Mix and set aside. May also purchase this blend from spice stores.

Mix 2 cans of chickpeas with olive oil in bowl. Preheat oven to 400. Place chickpeas evenly on a tray or platter and roast for about 30 minutes, stirring or shaking a few times to avoid browning too much.

Take out and let cool down. Sprinkle the spice blend and mix. May add a few drops of lemon juice for moisture and acidity. Great for a side dish or in a bean salad.

Nutrition Analysis:
Estimated per serving (1/2 of can): Calories 240; Protein 10 grams.

Portobello Mushroom Grill
Yield: 4 servings

Large, meaty Portobello mushrooms are juicy and flavorful. They can be baked as well as grilled, but grilling is my favorite way of preparing them. The stems are a bit tougher than the caps, but are good oiled and grilled next to them. The mushrooms are a terrific garnish for steak, roast chicken or turkey, or served with a salad for a meatless lunch. Any leftover mushrooms can be cut into pieces and served as a garnish for any meat or fish or added to a salad. They are also good mixed with eggs for an omelet or added to soups as an enhancement.

4 Large Portobello mushrooms, stems removed and reserved
    1 1/2 tbsp Good olive oil
    1/4 tsp Salt
    1/4 tsp Freshly ground black pepper

Heat a grill until very hot. Rub the top surface of the mushroom caps and the stems with the oil (which will be quickly absorbed) and sprinkle them with the salt and pepper. Place the caps top side down on the grill and cook, for about 3 minutes. Turn them over, and cook them for 3 minutes on the other side. Serve immediately, or set aside in a warm place until ready to serve.

As part of your meal plan, this recipe can be used as a side dish in a meal, in a salad or with eggs in the morning.

Nutrition Analysis:
Estimated per serving of about 62 grams: Calories 60, Protein 2 grams
Adapted from recipe by Jacques Pepin in *It Must Be My Metabolism* by R. Yavari, MD.

Iceberg Lettuce with Cucumber and Cannellini Bean Sauce
Serves 6

Ingredients

Cannellini Beans - 1 can (prefer organic), drained and rinsed
Iceberg Lettuce – Outer leaves removed, washed and drained
English Cucumber – 1 Peeled and sliced thin
Cilantro – 1 cup chopped
Flat Parsley – 1 cup chopped
Olive Oil – 2 tbsp
Hot Sauce – 1 tsp (your choice or omit)
Salt – 1 tsp
Black Pepper – 1 tsp
Garlic - 2 cloves, minced

Using a food processor, blend cilantro, parsley, garlic and olive oil for about 30 seconds, about 10 seconds at a time. Add beans and blend for an additional 30 seconds stopping every a few times to check if all ingredients are mixed well. Add salt, pepper and hot sauce to taste. Transfer to a bowl.

Cut iceberg lettuce into 6 wedges. Pour dip on wedges, add cucumber slices and serve.

Nutrition Analysis:
Estimated per serving: Calories 100; Protein 4 grams.

Baja Sauce

Ingredients

2 tbsp Chopped Red Bell Pepper (or ¼ of a pepper)
1   Chopped Jalapeno seeds and ribs removed
2 tbsp Chopped Red Onion
1 Clove Garlic minced
½ cup   Mayonnaise
½ cup   Sour cream or plain yogurt
1 tbsp Lime Juice
1 ts Honey
½ tsp   Cumin crushed
½ tsp   Salt
½ tsp Black pepper

Instructions

1. In the bowl of a food processor add all ingredients and pulse several times until well mixed.

2. Scrape down the sides of the bowl with a plastic spatula and blend till pureed.

3. Refrigerate for a few hours or overnight.

You may make more by doubling all ingredients – but may need a bigger blender.

Black Bean Salsa

Ingredients

2	Large Poblano peppers
2	Jalapeno peppers
1 or 2	Large red onion chopped into small squares
2 cloves	Fresh garlic minced
1 can	Organic cooked black Beans drained and rinsed
1 can	Organic diced tomato
2 tsp	Cumin seeds (crushed) or powder
2 tsp	Salt – may adjust to taste later

Juice of 2 Limes
Fresh Cilantro chopped
2 tbsp   Olive oil
1 cup   Vegetable Broth

Instructions

1. Cut peppers in halves lengthwise, remove seeds.
2. Roast in the oven at high temperature (450 +) for about 10 minutes or until skin browned.
3. Peel and chop peppers (remove skin in cold water – optional)
4. In a non-stick pan heat olive oil then add chopped onion, peppers and garlic.
5. Cook at medium temperature until onions are slightly translucent – do not brown.
6. Add dice tomatoes, mix.
7. Add black beans and mix.
8. Simmer in 1 cup of vegetable broth for about 15 minutes or until tomato pieces and beans are just soft.
9. Adjust salt.
10. Add lime juice and garnish with cilantro.

Cannellini Bean Dip

Ingredients

1 cup Fresh cilantro leaves (lightly packed)

3/4 cup Fresh parsley leaves (lightly packed)

3 cloves Garlic, peeled

1/2 tsp Salt

1/4 tsp Freshly ground black pepper

1   19-ounce can Cannelloni beans, drained

A few drops Tabasco hot pepper sauce

2 tbsp Extra virgin olive oil

Pita bread or toast

Instructions

Feel free to substitute another variety of canned beans—anything from black beans to red beans. You can serve the dip on cucumber slices or melba toasts instead of pita bread, if you prefer. This dip could also be used as a pasta sauce, extended with chicken stock for serving as a soup, or served lukewarm under a piece of poached codfish. As part of your meal plan, this recipe can be used as part of a meal, a salad or as a snack.

This recipe makes about 2 1/4 cups or about 7 servings.

1. Bring about 3 cups of water to a boil in a saucepan.

2. Add the cilantro and parsley and push the herbs down into the water.

3. Blanch for 10 seconds.

4. Drain the herbs in a sieve and spoon them into the bowl of a food processor.

5. Add the garlic, salt, and pepper, and process for a few seconds to combine the ingredients.

6. Add the drained beans and process for about 45 seconds, stopping the processor a few times and scraping down the sides of the bowl with a rubber spatula, until the mixture is smooth.

7. Add the Tabasco and olive oil, and process for about 5 seconds, until they are incorporated.

8. Transfer the bean dip to a serving bowl and serve with pita bread or toast.

Adapted from *It Must Be My Metabolism* by Reza Yavari, MD (recipe by Jacques Pepin)

Cucumber Yogurt Sauce

Ingredients

1 cup	Chopped cucumber (after peeling and removing seeds)
¼ cup	Chopped scallion
2 cloves	Chopped garlic
3 tbsp	Lime juice
1 tbsp	Olive oil
1.5 cups	Low-fat plain yogurt
2	Apples, peeled, cored and cut dice size
2.5 cups	Chopped mushrooms – Baby Bellas or button
1 tbsp	Fresh tarragon
½ tsp	Salt

Instructions

1. Put all the ingredients for the dressing, except the yogurt, in a blender, and blend until smooth.

2. Transfer the mixture to a bowl and stir in the yogurt. (You will have about 2 cups.)

3. Set aside or refrigerator for up to 10 days to use on salads or grilled meat or fish.

Adapted from *It Must Be My Metabolism* by Reza Yavari, MD (recipe by Jacques Pepin)

Fresh Tomato Salsa
Ingredients
1 can (15oz)   Diced Glen-Muir tomatoes or similar
1   Jalapeno, chopped, seeds and ribs removed
½ medium   Chopped red onion
3 tbsp   Chopped cilantro
½ tsp   Salt
Instructions
1. Add ingredients to a blender and pulse a few times to mix well but not pureed.
2. Set aside or refrigerate for later use.

You could make more by doubling all ingredients.
Instructions
1. Add ingredients to a blender and pulse a few times to mix well but not pureed.
2. Set aside or refrigerate for later use.

You could make more by doubling all ingredients.

Hummus Homemade

Ingredients

1 can	Chickpeas (prefer organic), drained and rinsed
3-4 tbsp	Tahini
2 cloves	Garlic, chopped and pressed
1 tbsp	Olive oil
2 tbsp	Lemon juice
¼ cup	Water
1 tsp	Salt

Instructions

Hummus is now widely available in all sizes and flavors. However, it is east to make at home and ingredients such as tahini, garlic, oil and salt and water could be adjusted to taste.

1. Add all ingredients to a blender and add ½ of water.
2. Pulse till well mixed.
3. Add the remainder of water and pulse a few more times.
4. Taste and adjust oil and salt if needed.

You could make more by doubling all ingredients.

Mango Salsa

Ingredients

1	Chopped Mango
1	Jalapeno, chopped, seeds and ribs removed
1 medium	Chopped red onion
2 Tbsp.	Chopped cilantro
2 Tbsp.	Lime juice
½ Tsp.	Salt
½ Tsp.	Sugar

Instructions

1. Mix all ingredients well.
2. Set aside at room temperature or keep in refrigerator for later use.

You could make more by doubling every ingredient.

Sofrito

Ingredients

2 Tbsp.	Olive oil
4	Green peppers, seeds and ribs removed
2	Red Bell peppers, seeds and ribs removed
2 large	Tomatoes, cut
2 medium	Chopped onions
2 cloves	Chopped garlic
1 batch	Chopped cilantro
½ tsp	Salt

Instructions

1. Place all ingredients together in a blender to puree.
2. Pour into small containers and keep frozen till ready to use.

RESOURCES

AVAILABLE ON AMAZON and other bookstores:

- *It Must Be My Metabolism*

Reza Yavari, MD

- *Simulation Coaching for Obesity & Diabetes*

Reza Yavari, MD

Available online:

- *Beyond Weight Coaching App*

Find out more at www.beyondweight.com

Made in the USA
Middletown, DE
10 November 2022